Quality Assisted Living

Leslie A. Morgan, PhD, is Professor of Sociology and Co-director of the Doctoral Program in Gerontology at University of Maryland, Baltimore County (UMBC). An affiliate of the Center for Aging Studies, she has authored or co-authored five books and over 30 journal articles on topics relating to family, senior housing, economics, and gender. She is a fellow of the Gerontological Society of America and of the Association for Gerontology in Higher Education.

Ann Christine Frankowski, PhD, a cultural anthropologist, is Associate Research Scientist in the Department of Sociology and Anthropology, University of Maryland, Baltimore County (UMBC), conducting ethnographic studies at its Center for Aging Studies. She is co-author of *Inside Assisted Living* and articles on sociocultural aspects of senior housing.

Erin G. Roth, MA, is a Senior Research Analyst and Ethnographer with the Center for Aging Studies at University of Maryland, Baltimore County (UMBC). Trained as a folklorist, she worked in the public sector prior to joining the Center in 2004. She is a co-author of *Inside Assisted Living* and has contributed articles to the *Journal of Aging Studies*, the *Journal of American Folklore*, and the *Journal of Folklore Research*.

Lynn Keimig, MHA, PhD candidate, has worked as Project Coordinator on two studies related to assisted living and currently is part of the research team for two studies, focusing on social stigma in senior housing and generativity in later life, in the Center for Aging Studies at University of Maryland, Baltimore County (UMBC). Her own research focuses on family structure and advance care planning.

Sheryl Zimmerman, PhD, is Kenan Distinguished Professor and Director of Aging Research, School of Social Work and Co-director, Program on Aging, Disability, and Long-Term Care, Cecil G. Sheps Center for Health Services Research, University of North Carolina at Chapel Hill. Dr. Zimmerman has been a consulting social worker in nursing homes and assisted living facilities. She has led widely disseminated research on quality of care and quality of life, involving thousands of long-term care residents and the family and staff who provide their care.

J. Kevin Eckert, PhD, is Professor and Chair of the Department of Sociology and Anthropology at University of Maryland, Baltimore County (UMBC). An affiliate of the Center for Aging Studies, he has been a lead investigator on several studies and published widely on topics relating to the experience of older adults living in age-restricted housing and care settings. He is a fellow of the Gerontological Society of America and of the Association for Gerontology in Higher Education.

Quality Assisted Living

Informing Practice Through Research

Leslie A. Morgan, PhD
Ann Christine Frankowski, PhD
Erin G. Roth, MA
Lynn Keimig, MHA
Sheryl Zimmerman, PhD
J. Kevin Eckert, PhD

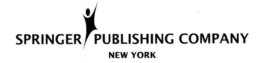

SPRINGER PUBLISHING COMPANY
NEW YORK

Springer Publishing Company, LLC
11 West 42nd Street
New York, NY 10036
www.springerpub.com

Acquisitions Editor: Sheri W. Sussman
Senior Production Editor: Diane Davis
Composition: NewGen Imaging

ISBN: 978-0-8261-3034-1
E-book ISBN: 978-0-8261-3035-8

11 12 13 14 15 16   5 4 3 2 1

The author and the publisher of this Work have made every effort to use sources believed to be reliable to provide information that is accurate and compatible with the standards generally accepted at the time of publication. Because medical science is continually advancing, our knowledge base continues to expand. Therefore, as new information becomes available, changes in procedures become necessary. We recommend that the reader always consult current research and specific institutional policies before performing any clinical procedure. The author and publisher shall not be liable for any special, consequential, or exemplary damages resulting, in whole or in part, from the readers' use of, or reliance on, the information contained in this book. The publisher has no responsibility for the persistence or accuracy of URLs for external or third-party Internet Web sites referred to in this publication and does not guarantee that any content on such Web sites is, or will remain, accurate or appropriate.

Library of Congress Cataloging-in-Publication Data
Quality assisted living : informing practice through research / Leslie A. Morgan...[et al.].
    p. cm.
  Includes bibliographical references and index.
  ISBN 978-0-8261-3034-1—ISBN 978-0-8261-3035-8 (ebook)
  1. Old age homes. 2. Nursing homes. 3. Congregate housing. 4. Older people—Care.
I. Morgan, Leslie A.
  HV1454.Q35 2011
  362.61—dc22   2011015449

Special discounts on bulk quantities of our books are available to corporations, professional associations, pharmaceutical companies, health care organizations, and other qualifying groups.

If you are interested in a custom book, including chapters from more than one of our titles, we can provide that service as well.

For details, please contact:
Special Sales Department, Springer Publishing Company, LLC
11 West 42nd Street, 15th Floor, New York, NY 10036—8002
Phone: 877-687-7476 or 212-431-4370; Fax: 212-941-7842
Email: sales@springerpub.com

Printed in the United States of America by Gasch Printing.

Contents

Preface

Concern regarding quality in assisted living (AL) is well established. All 50 states regulate the care settings they label as "assisted living" in order to minimize risks to safety and guarantee a basic set of rights and services to residents (Mollica, Sims-Kastelein, & O'Keefe, 2007). Provider organizations, such as Leading Age and the Assisted Living Federation of America, and advocacy groups like the Center for Excellence in Assisted Living spend considerable time focusing on how to create, improve, and sustain quality in their settings, both in serving the goals of their businesses and as providers of housing and care for residents. With some regularity, journalists uncover stories of shockingly poor care, neglect, abuse, or unnecessary death in AL; similar stories have, over decades, resulted in today's high level of regulation and oversight of nursing homes (Kane, 2010). Although regulations provide an acceptable basic level of housing and care while working to avoid the most egregious types of abuse or neglect, the question of reaching a fuller and more responsive level of quality remains unaddressed.

One key factor in the puzzle of understanding quality is determining what matters most and to whom it matters: the regulators, operators and managers, direct care providers, or residents and family members. Whereas managers and owners must be responsive to the goals of regulators or the external marketplace, people living in AL bring experiences and expectations for their housing and care, which shape the dimensions that matter most to quality. The study that serves as the primary basis of this book focuses specifically on the problem of gaining a deeper understanding of the meaning of quality from the perspective of people living and working in AL. As researchers, we have found that our views of what constitutes quality aren't always shared by those living or working there. We found that a "one-size-fits-all" idea about what AL settings offer or about what residents or their kin are seeking when in search of services to be equally unrealistic. Details about the research process are included in the Appendix.

Based in our research team's prior work in AL, we saw many family and staff members, leaders and managers, and residents who expressed concerns about—or praised aspects of—their life or work in AL. We also learned from experiences in a variety of AL settings that quality may be difficult to discern, hidden in the mundane daily routines of life, such as meals, activities, room cleaning, and interactions with others in the setting. Our observations also showed that our views about what made for a good quality setting weren't always mirrored by those to whom we spoke, suggesting that quality is, perhaps, more complicated than the simple researcher checklists or customer satisfaction surveys that have been employed to gauge quality to date.

Our collaborative research team, including the listed authors and two other important colleagues (Robert L. Rubinstein and Leanne Clark-Shirley), spent considerable time together discussing and debating the varied ideas coming from our groups of interviewees. In doing so, we learned a great deal about how life unfolds in AL and about some of the challenges faced by this sector as it matures and addresses the aging in place of residents and deals with the economic downturn that started in 2008.

Leslie A. Morgan

REFERENCES

Kane, R. T. (2010). Reimagining Nursing Homes: The Art of the Possible. *Journal of Aging & Social Policy*, 22(4), 321–333.

Mollica, R., Sims-Kastelein, K., & O'Keefe, J. (2007). *Residential Care and Assisted Living Compendium: 2007*. Received from http://aspe.hhs.gov/daltcp/reports/2007/07alcom.htm

Acknowledgments

We would like to acknowledge the support of NIA in funding "Stakeholders' Models of Quality in Assisted Living" (1 R01 AG022563, Leslie A. Morgan, PI). We also appreciate the supportive environments of our academic institutions (University of Maryland, Baltimore County and University of North Carolina, Chapel Hill), as well as our more extended network of colleagues. Our greatest gratitude is to the assisted living settings, managers, staff, residents, and family members who gave us their valuable time for the interviews that have revealed the insights included in this book. They are the true experts on assisted living, and have taught us many important lessons through their involvement in our work.

1
Quality in Assisted Living
Hearing Residents' Voices

ORIENTING POINTS

- Current means of evaluating quality focus on priorities of groups other than assisted living residents.
- Quality is subjective and relative to the resident's experiences and expectations.
- Quality priorities vary among residents and differ from the views of other assisted living participants.

WHAT IS QUALITY?

The dramatic growth of the assisted living (AL) sector has generated a substantial interest in evaluating and enhancing its quality. While early examinations by researchers and policy analysts generated information on the characteristics of AL settings, services, staff, and residents (Hawes, Rose, & Phillips, 1999; Zimmerman, Sloane, & Eckert, 2001), limited attention has addressed the distinct dimensions of quality in AL, particularly in contrast to aspects prominent in nursing homes. Although everyone wants to foster or find quality in AL, the question remains: What exactly is quality? It is a question of clear interest to the older adults residing and receiving services in ALs, as well as to their family members or advocates, AL providers, and staff members. The purpose of this book is to explore the meanings of quality, focusing most centrally on the views and voices of those who, we argue, matter most—the older adults who reside in AL settings 24 hours a day, 7 days a week.

This book examines AL quality from the ground up by focusing on the views of older adults who reside in seven AL settings about what matters most to them in their daily lives. Views of these day-to-day participants are less visible in current quality discussions, which more often attend to the priorities of regulators, academic researchers, or corporate owners, rather than those of individuals living, visiting, or working daily in AL. What precisely are the meanings intended when a staff person, a family member, or a resident describes a setting as being of good or poor quality? The word *quality* is quite broad, carrying a positive implication; yet in discussion we sometimes use it as though we have a clear and, most importantly, a *shared* perspective on what makes for a "high-quality" AL setting. We contend in this book that quality, like many other evaluative judgments, arises from the perspective and framework of expectations and experience of the beholder; consequently, opinions about quality vary widely among individuals residing in AL and also differ from views of other groups, like kin, staff, managers, or regulators.

Views of Quality: The Resident Quality Balance

From the perspective of residents, quality can be viewed as a personal balance, which is dynamic through time, rather than as a fixed, standard checklist capturing widely shared views. There are two sides to this balance—the profile of the resident and that of the AL setting. Key to achieving a quality balance for a given resident is the degree of match between his or her profile, composed of the residents' experiences, needs, wants, and preferences, against the profile of setting, including aspects of staffing and services provided by the AL. An optimal situation is achieved when there is a balance between these two profiles, as shown in Figure 1.1. Varying degrees of imbalance, resulting in a moderate or large movement of the arrowhead away from the center point of peak quality, lead to an experience of lower quality.

This quality balance concept builds upon the idea of person/environment fit, which has long been discussed as essential for older adults in any housing environment (Lawton & Nahemow, 1975). The focus on fit traditionally emphasized how aging persons change, resulting in their environments becoming less suitable, and mirroring discussions of AL conditions, which have focused on changes in residents and largely neglected changes in AL settings as important to quality

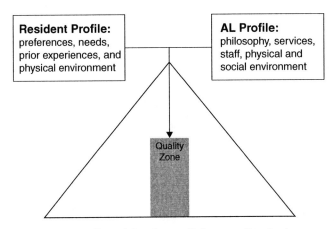

Figure 1.1. Graphic view of the quality balance.

(Ball et al., 2004). Instead, this model implies that change on either or both sides of the quality balance may result in an improved or diminished quality experience for residents. Since not all residents emphasize the same elements as priorities in assessing quality, and each AL provides a distinct environment and culture of service, the inadequacy of "one size fits all" definitions quickly becomes apparent.

Quality, as we uncovered it, is achieved (or approached) when what a person residing in AL seeks in terms of a physical environment (building, location, room, and accessibility); needs for care (medication, oversight, and assistance); and prefers (flexibility, privacy, and social engagement) is matched by what the AL offers. To the degree there is a mismatch, a small or larger imbalance will occur, sometimes moving beyond the boundaries of the quality zone. The most often recognized imbalance in this equation is when a resident's needs for medical or personal care outweigh the capacity of the AL to meet them. However, imbalances occur for many other reasons.

Consequently, quality, based on the resident's view, is not comprised of a single, uniform checklist of items to be achieved by an AL's management and staff. Instead, quality occurs when there is a balance, to be approached or achieved for each place and relative to each resident within it. Customers seeking AL services attempt to locate this balance through the selection of the "right place" for a given person, insofar as they understand the profile of the future resident and can discover that of the AL. For example, some residents prefer a smaller-scale

AL setting, with a more physically and socially intimate environment; others prefer larger, more bustling places that provide a variety of people, activities, and spaces. But, there are elements of the AL profile that are not immediately visible or easily understood during visits and tours. And, even if the profiles of person and place are balanced when a new resident arrives, it is common for this balance to change over time. Either a resident's profile may change or important changes in the AL, which will be discussed in Chapter 7, will alter the quality balance. This view of the quality balance represents a key challenge for the AL sector, as it requires individual providers to meet diverse needs, preferences, and goals for those living and receiving care there while operating within state regulations and with limited resources.

Because the quality balance includes a number of moving parts, it provides daily opportunities for quality to be evaluated by residents and other participants in the setting. Everyday encounters between persons and places (or the people in them, such as staff members) may lead to shifting quality evaluations. An embarrassing or uplifting encounter with a direct care worker, for example, may alter a resident's view of quality. Thus, from a single incident the resident's balance may tilt one way or another, shifting the evaluation into or out of the quality zone. In this chapter, we discuss how elements of the quality profile vary across different residents, and how resident priorities do not entirely coincide with those of their kin, AL staff members and providers, or regulators, although there is often considerable overlap. In several of the following chapters, perspectives of other groups are included, showing these differences in perspectives on quality.

The Study

Although there is a lot of discussion about AL quality, the intention of the 4-year study that provides the data for this book was to examine what people *mean* when they think of or talk about quality—in other words, what are the elements upon which a quality evaluation is built? Rather than assuming we knew what makes for a "good quality" experience, our study took quality as something to be uncovered and better understood through careful interviewing, allowing the participants to identify what mattered most to them. Although many AL settings routinely performed customer satisfaction surveys or gather feedback at meetings of a Resident Council or similar group, some participants withheld their concerns, voicing them only to peers or family members rather than to staff or managers. Others were quite vocal, viewing themselves as AL consumers with the right to get what they paid for.

This research was conducted in seven AL settings in Maryland, identified as demonstrating the diversity that exists in this housing and care sector in aspects such as size, for-profit or nonprofit status, being (or not being) part of a chain, religious affiliation/sponsorship, resident race/ethnicity profile, as well as location in suburban, or rural areas—several adjacent to large urban centers. Table 1.1 identifies these participating settings by their pseudonyms, which will be used in the chapters to follow. In each of these settings, we conducted in-depth interviews with 10–12 older adults residing there, a similar number of their family members or advocates, five direct care staff members, and up to three administrators or managers.

When we interviewed family members of residents (or those undertaking kin-like responsibilities), direct care staff, and administrators/managers, we used parallel questions to those for residents, asking questions such as what makes for a good or bad day *for residents,* or what changes they would suggest if they were in charge or were building an entirely new AL. The questions offered multiple opportunities for people in each group to identify things that mattered to them—in

Table 1.1.   Characteristics of AL Settings

Pseudonym	No. of Beds	Chain?	Profit Status	Location	Religious	% Non-White
Boxwood Gardens	104	Yes	For-profit	Suburban	No	14
St. Brigid	18	No	Nonprofit	Suburban	Yes	10
Murray Ridge	36	No	For-profit	Rural	No	0
Wetherby Place	48	Yes	Nonprofit	Suburban	Yes	3
Greenbriar	92	Yes	For-profit	Suburban	No	75
Arcadia Springs	45	No	For-profit	Suburban	No	9
Winter Hills	75	Yes	For-profit	Rural	No	0

short, their bases of quality in AL life for residents. The research team then analyzed the themes and meanings related to quality from audiotaped interviews and built a database of the interviews, which was coded to enable us to identify material relating to key themes or to search for connections among themes and across interviews and groups. Most of the codes we used to tag quotations appearing here arose from interviews with residents, with a few added from family and AL staff/administrator interviews. These codes helped us to explore, compare, and connect the ideas within and across interviews.

In a second step of the study, we took key concepts from interviews and asked all participants to rate their importance by sorting cards with these themes printed on them into piles of most important, important, or not important to themselves (residents), to residents (staff/administrators), or to their relatives (family). Residents were assisted by researchers in this task through reading or handling of cards, if needed. Results of this card sorting task will be described further later in this chapter.

One essential goal in conducting our study was to ensure that everyone being interviewed understood that what they told us was confidential and we were not conducting quality assessment for the AL setting. In a few cases, residents declined to have their interviews audiotaped, because of the concerns that someone beyond our research team might learn of negative aspects of AL life revealed in their interviews. Following rules of research, we reassured participants of confidentiality but accepted their wishes not to answer some of our questions or to reveal some stories of life in AL. It appears that concerns about disclosing negative views were an extension of a generalized worry that complaining might bring trouble, a topic addressed further in coming chapters. Although most information comes from interviews at the seven sites discussed previously, this research team has conducted research in two other studies.[1] Some examples from these projects are included here as well.

---

[1] The first grant was "Transitions from Assisted Living: Sociocultural Factors." NIA Grant, (J. Kevin Eckert P.I.) The second project, "Social Relations in Residential Care," NIA Grant (J. Kevin Eckert P.I.) is ongoing as of this writing.

Understanding the Complexity of Quality

Although we generally think that many people would share similar definitions of quality, our interviews revealed a great deal of complexity and diversity in the criteria upon which residents based their views. Quality was, in short, in the eye of the beholder. What may represent good quality for one resident may not be good for another, and what one resident deems as central within the housing and services of AL also may differ notably from the priorities of the employee who helps her dress in the morning or her own family members. This diversity was demonstrated across numerous residents we interviewed, including a medical man with multiple health problems, Dr. Styles. Dr. Styles said, comparing the Greenbriar and other ALs, "*I think each Assisted Living area is going to satisfy a certain social group. They're not all going to be satisfying to the same group. I mean it's like housing—some people are going to want to live in a certain area with certain things—and others don't give a damn.*" Similarly, Mr. Leland, resident of the nonprofit St. Brigid, said, "*It's hard to define quality really. Depends on how you look at it on a certain time, certain part of the day. Sometimes it's good, sometimes it's bad—you know? It really is hard to tell.*"

This complexity of quality is encountered daily by providers when activities they offer are enjoyed by some but don't suit others or when physical amenities, such as nicely decorated public areas that may please a family member, seem irrelevant to the resident, her father, who instead cares mostly about the staff available for 24-hour health oversight or about the privacy of his room. Agencies across the states that regulate AL settings are likely to include one set of items on their checklists of quality, whereas those living, visiting, or working inside these settings may include very different priorities about what makes for high quality.

In short, the term "quality" is a broad generality that really does not tell us what matters on a day-to-day basis for any specific person within the walls of any AL setting. The viewpoint that has been most neglected is that of the individuals residing in AL, whose 24/7 exposure to the setting provides a distinct perspective. It is the views of these residents that serve as the central focus for this book. To readily distinguish the residents' personal insights regarding life in an AL setting from those provided by family members, visitors, and AL staff, we have set off the residents' replies to our research team's inquiries in italics.

Diverse Resident Perspectives on Quality

A good starting point in understanding resident perspectives on quality is to contrast the views of three women residing in the same setting during our months of research there. From one view, what these individuals experience is largely the same. They have access to the same activities, are located in the same community, are served the same meals, and share a staff, a single leadership philosophy, and a physical environment. But, as their descriptions make clear, residents' views of what mattered within AL differed.

Jean Thompson: Visiting—"It's not like being a resident."

After nearly a year, Jean Thompson was adjusting fairly well to her routine at Murray Ridge, where she had moved after a year-long stay at a nursing home/rehabilitation center where she was sent to address multiple health problems. Having had a cousin who previously lived there, she said that Murray Ridge was *"pretty much…what I thought it would be."* She liked many things about her assisted living, including having a private room, so that she could keep to herself when she wished. She also said that she liked the food, the grounds which were shaded by surrounding trees, and the staff, for carefully attending to cleanliness and the *"little things."* Especially important to Ms. Thompson was the fact that the staff knew each person as an individual. *"[I]t's sort of knowing your residents, concern for individuals, knowing their tastes, what they like or dislike, are important considerations."* She attended some of the activities and was still able to pursue her lifelong pattern of reading every day, developed while she was a teacher and librarian, with ample books available from the visiting Bookmobile.

Ms. Thompson was working on getting used to being dependent on others, saying, *"[I]t's the idea you have to depend on somebody—if I go out, I got to depend on somebody else to take me. It's sort of a loss of independence. I think that's the hardest thing for me."* While she was working on accepting her dependence and was positive about Murray Ridge, there was still room for improvement, in her view. She noted problems with staff shortages, when workers were *"not showing up for their shift."*

Ms. Thompson brought with her both her own experience in a nursing home prior to moving into Murray Ridge and earlier experiences that stuck with her. *"We took care of my mother at home until she was in her last illness and she was in a nursing home about five months. But that's not like being a resident. Then my elderly uncle was in a nursing home for almost a year. But it still—even if you go and you try to help…it's not like being a resident. Well, you have a different outlook, you come and go. It's just different."* Ms. Thompson was clear that her perspective changed when she moved from the role of a visiting family member to a full-time resident of assisted living.

Millie Fischer: "It's not home, but it's nice."

Downstairs from Jean Thompson at Murray Ridge, Millie Fischer chose to reside in the small dementia care unit, even though she was "eligible" to reside in the general care unit upstairs. She preferred the smaller dementia unit, which limited her exposure to the unwelcome realities of life upstairs—in particular the fact that she was living with people other than her family. Having worked as a nurse, Ms. Fischer said that Murray Ridge was "a regular nursing home," with both good (e.g., having people to help) and bad aspects that went with such a setting (e.g., boredom and insufficient staff). *"Well, it's a place where they're supposed to take care of you."*

A woman of few words, Ms. Fischer was clear that Murray Ridge was not acceptable for her, even if it was nice for other people. When asked what would make for a good day for her, her terse answer was to *"go home,"* explaining later that what had been important in her life has been *"just being with my family."* She had few specific suggestions on how to improve things at Murray Ridge, except to have staff spend more time talking with "patients" about things, including their families. After giving her AL a grade of 75 (because *"nothing's perfect"*), Millie summed up her feelings by saying, *"It's a nice place to live. It's not home, but it's nice."* Asked if there was any way to make it home for her she replied, *"You can't [have a home] without your family."*

Eileen Howe: "It's what we make it."

Ms. Howe took the attitude that life is what you make it in AL. *"It's what we make it, you know what I mean. You want to be a grouch, you want to complain—there's really nothing to complain about. . . . We just have become one family. You know, we hear bad news and somebody's family sick, we all care. It's made us—it's made us—we'll be friends forever. I can't explain it. Nobody is stuck up."* She compiled quite a list of things she liked, including *"it's kept clean, we have privacy. During the night, nobody is coming in the room scaring you half to death,"* and *"they see that we play bingo a couple times and we sit in the sitting room, some times and just talk. And honestly it's really—I can't say enough for it. . . . I'm very happy here. Because I'm not lonesome, and everybody here is—I think if you weren't nice, maybe they wouldn't let you stay here, I don't know. But nobody gets in arguments, because that would scare me."* While claiming it's not fancy and would not fit for everyone, Ms. Howe said, *"I just—it's home. I don't know whether everybody feels like that here, but it just is—with me, I've made it home."* When asked near the end of her interview to identify her three favorite things about living at Murray Ridge, she said, *"I love the privacy that we have. Our meals are very good—most of all I like it because it becomes home. Doesn't seem like an institution, you know. . . ."*

Although these women lived in the same AL, they each viewed it differently, based on their varied priorities and goals. Their views also diverged from those of the director. When Darlene Hall, a local girl who had essentially grown up working at Murray Ridge and now ran its day-to-day operations for private owners, was asked about what makes for a good day for the people living there, her answer was clear.

> Good day for a resident? . . . . If they're going to get out of the bed. Because we have some residents who just want to lay in their—sit in their room. So if they get out of the bed, you know wake up in the morning, get dressed, eat their breakfast, stay out of the room and do the activities, eat all their meals and then you know go into their room at night time, or evening after dinner then they get ready for bed. A lot of them want to stay in their room and not socialize, so a good day would be for them to get out and socialize and do the activities. Which most of them do now.

Her ideas about AL quality, focusing on a functional daily routine and her belief that social activities were good for everyone, grew directly out of her predecessor's philosophy. While Ms. Howe might endorse Darlene's agenda, Ms. Thompson clearly valued her privacy and having quiet time alone to read over attending all activities. Ms. Fischer rejected the activities and socializing altogether by choosing to live downstairs, away from the people and social contact of the AL community. Quality of daily life was defined for her solely by what was absent in AL—her family. Clearly, these residents saw aspects for a good (or bad) day in AL that differed in some notable ways from manager Darlene's quality priorities.

Understanding Quality: Key Questions

Expecting that each individual involved in AL could, with modest reflection, generate a list of items that they would employ as the basis for quality evaluations, our interviewers asked what participants thought mattered most on a day-to-day basis. We'll begin our discussion of the complex results of these interviews by employing five main questions. First, is AL quality more about the quality of daily life or the quality of the care that people receive? For nursing homes this answer is clearly oriented toward health care; for AL the answer remains unsettled, particularly since the residents age in place and may need more health services over time (Ball et al., 2004; Zimmerman et al., 2003). Second, how many pieces are there to the quality puzzle? Do all individuals have a large list of items that matter to them in assessing quality, or do some focus on only a few, pivotal elements in evaluating AL quality? The third question addresses the reference point for quality: Quality compared to what? Our interviews identified a number of concrete reference points, including one's prior home, earlier care settings for oneself or others, or current alternatives. The fourth question asks whose viewpoint on quality we should favor: should resident views or those of family or expert professionals influence AL priorities? This question becomes moot if all parties share a common view of what makes for good quality, but becomes increasingly important if priorities for quality differ across groups. This issue of consensus (or its absence) can be a key to addressing the challenge of quality. The fifth question, introduced here but discussed more fully in Chapter 7, is whether and how quality changes over time and the role of the AL setting in altering the quality equation through its own changes. If the balance between person and place is essential to quality outcomes, changes in either could diminish that fit, resulting in poorer quality. We address each of the first four questions in turn.

Question 1: Quality of Life or Quality of Care: Is AL Quality About Health Care?

As this new housing sector was emerging, its advocates worked to distinguish AL from nursing homes. The keystone of that difference was the social model of care, focusing more on quality of life, in contrast to nursing homes' medical model, which primarily addresses the quality of health care and services (Wilson, 1990). While acknowledging that most people move into AL for health-related reasons, AL advocates identified its mission as providing personal care and assistance within a supportive living environment (including meals and cleaning services); promoters drew a line, eventually reinforced by state regulations, limiting how much "medical care" a resident can require before he or she must leave AL (Mollica, Sims-Kastelein, & O'Keefe, 2007). In short, the mission of AL at its outset focused more on quality of life than on quality of care issues. In examining our resident interviews, however, we found a mixture of quality of life along with quality of care elements among their priorities; some focused on only one, whereas many others combined elements of both dimensions.

Although choice and autonomy are among the quality of life goals in the social model of care, not all of the residents prioritized them. Ms. Teiman emphasized quality of health care and oversight in her interview, even if it meant fewer choices for herself and her peers living at Boxwood Gardens—for their own good. She described her AL as just like a nursing home, with "*stroke patients and drooling, depressed people, people that had oxygen around their neck.*" She complained both about the inadequate staff-to- "patient" ratio at Boxwood Gardens as well as the lack of strict dietary enforcement for diabetics like herself. Hoping to move soon, when asked what she'd look for in another AL, Ms. Teiman said, "*... the ratio of help they have according to the number of people that live there. One nurse for 25 patients doesn't cut the mustard with me....People that are supposed to be around at 1:00 o'clock in the morning are what I care about.*"

Ms. Carson, a very vocal interviewee with multiple concerns, when asked what would make life nicer or better for people living at Boxwood Gardens said, "*Oh, my—well, I have thought to myself, and said to myself sometimes they are trying to do an impossible job. The first thing I would do would be to get a medical doctor in and nurses who are working with the doctors, happily—and are allowed to work as nurses. I'd get a nutritionist who is not working for some contracted food company. In other words, I would look at health and medicine and I would include psychological care.*"

In contrast, Ms. Stone, who continued to attend her own church every Sunday, using a car and driver hired by her son, focused primarily on the social aspects of life at the Greenbriar. Responding to the question of what made for a good day for her, Ms. Stone described an active social agenda.

> **Ms. Stone:** *Well, a good day—we play bingo twice a week. We play Pokeno—once a week, and—now Tuesdays I, which I call my off days, I catch up on my correspondence. Now, I get a lot of phone calls.*
>
> **Researcher:** You do?
>
> **Ms. Stone:** *'Cause my children call me all the time. I am not—I don't feel alone. And I can satisfy myself with the TV. I have a lot of TV shows that I like, and I do look at them. I just don't get lonesome. We were talking about that the other day, about being lonesome.*
>
> **Researcher:** Some of the residents were talking about that?
>
> **Ms. Stone:** *Oh, yeah. It was a topic of discussion—loneliness. But I haven't—I just haven't come into that . . . .*

Martha Harding considers it a blessing to live in her religiously focused setting, which enables her to attend Mass daily and visit the chapel 24 hours a day. She likes almost all of the other people living at St. Brigid except one "grouch," and has accepted changes, such as the director removing from her room a favorite rocking chair and throw rugs that were deemed to present a risk for falling. Like Ms. Stone, she found most of her satisfaction from the social aspects of AL, but Ms. Harding also valued the health care, recounting an emergency she had faced.

> *I started vomiting. And when I did, my friend that was here, she immediately called the nurse. And in a split second almost there were*

two nurses in here. And one says to the other, "Bring two pillows in here."...Anyway, it was like angels that suddenly appeared. And they took real good care of me and within the next day, I was pretty good. I can't remember why it happened. I don't remember, but that shows you—really, [they] may not always be able to get here when they don't have a nurse on the schedule...but they try to have a nurse all the time on duty, even though this is assisted living.

In short, while quality of care may be a major focus for regulators, staff, and administrators, many residents include substantial quality of life considerations in their views of what is important to a good life in AL.

Question 2: How Many Pieces in the Quality Puzzle?

In our interviews, residents identified many aspects of AL life that mattered to them in determining quality. In some cases, there was one central theme or topic in the interview, such as the AL's activities or their room's privacy, which served as the focus; for others, such as Ms. Morris from Boxwood Gardens, we came away with a laundry list of positive and negative elements that were important to her. Wheelchair bound due to a stroke, her initial reply about what made for a good day for her in AL did not relate to the AL, per se.

Ms. Morris: *When my daughter comes over to see me.*

Researcher: That makes a good day?

Ms. Morris: *Or friends come over and they do.*

Researcher: Do you have a lot of friends in the neighborhood?

Ms. Morris: *No. My coworkers come by.*

Researcher: Oh, that's nice.

Ms. Morris: *And my daughters come by and I have a special friend from [nearby town] almost every day.*

Ms. Morris raised many other issues during her interview. She liked Boxwood Gardens, noting it was kept clean and that people (both staff and residents) got along well. She described in particular enjoyment of the dining experience with a favorite dining partner, sharing humor as well as food. She also enjoyed scheduled activities, particularly trips outside the AL, but thought the music programs were poor and that there weren't enough other activities. When asked what made for a day that was not good, her reply was clear, *"Nothing to do. Just sitting around—I can't stand that, just sitting around."*

Identifying what she would do differently if she ran Boxwood Gardens, Ms. Morris's answers focused on staffing and health services. One health care dimension was lacking in her view. *"I would have in-house—plenty of [physical] therapy."* In addition, she shared concerns about adequate levels of staffing that were common to many residents we interviewed.

> **Ms. Morris:** *I would make sure that people didn't have off on the weekends. No weekends off—our weekends are very short [of staff].*
>
> **Researcher:** So you're short staffed on the weekends?
>
> **Ms. Morris:** *Yeah, always. I'd schedule all of them on weekends.*

In contrast to Ms. Morris, some individuals had just one central element identified as essential to quality or a good day in AL. Frank Trickett of Arcadia Springs, when asked if there was anything he didn't like, said, *"Well, I don't know of anything."* His very limited and repetitive interview responses may indicate some memory issues. Led through his busy days by a "bossy" female companion, his interview focused only on activities, in which he fully participated every day.

> **Researcher:** I noticed that you write down the day's activities on a card that you keep in your pocket.
>
> **Mr. Trickett:** *Yeah, right.*
>
> **Researcher:** Just so you know what's coming up.
>
> **Mr. Trickett:** *So I know what's going on, right. Got this one right here, if you can read it.*
>
> **Researcher [reading]:** 10:30 is exercise and 1:00 o'clock is volleyball, 2:00 o'clock is the short stories. 2:30, what does that say? Oh you said something about questions—
>
> **Mr. Trickett:** *Twenty Questions. 5:00 o'clock is Book Club.*
>
> **Researcher:** Book Club. What are you reading for the Book Club?
>
> **Mr. Trickett:** *Oh, I don't know.*

> *Researcher:* Do you go to everything?
>
> *Mr. Trickett: Well, yeah I go to the activities, yeah.*

Mr. Trickett also briefly mentioned that staff members were nice and *"help you when they can,"* but the bulk of the interview focused on the busy schedule of daily activities offered at Arcadia Springs.

> *Mr. Trickett: Well, it's a nice place... good place. Lot of stuff going on you know and interesting things. Got a regular agenda every day, so it keeps you busy.*
>
> *Researcher:* And that's what you were looking for in some place.
>
> *Mr. Trickett: Yeah, right, right.*

Beyond these extremes, the residents interviewed presented a wide array of topics as central elements for making daily life good or bad in their particular AL setting. In analyzing the interview transcripts, we found that several broad topics, such as traits and behaviors of the AL staff or food and dining issues, were addressed in more detailed ways by interviewees than might be indicated in simple questions of "How is the food?" or "How well do staff members care for you?" For example, eight codes emerged from resident interviews that related to the AL's physical environment. These included accessibility issues (elevators, ease of moving around, wheelchair access, etc.), the ambiance or "feel" of the place (i.e., hominess), furnishings (quality of one's own or the AL's furniture, fixtures), the nature/ quality of outdoor spaces and outdoor views, the capacity to have privacy, the AL's proximity to kin and other important people or places, the qualities of public spaces (size, furnishings, lighting, and usage), and the adequacy of one's own room/suite (e.g., its size, layout, and storage). With over 50 coding categories developed to capture elements from the interviews, the resident priorities represent both expected and unexpected elements that matter to at least some of the interviewees. Seemingly straightforward and open questions, asking what makes for good and bad days, what they would change if they ran the AL, or things that make for quality, generated a rich listing of elements among each of our four groups (residents, family, direct care staff, and managers), which serve as the underpinnings for their evaluations of quality.

Similar complexity was uncovered in other areas, such as attitudes and behaviors of direct care staff or opportunities for autonomy in daily life. Mr. Levenson, a diabetic double amputee who described himself as "hell bent" on learning to walk with his prostheses, focused much of his concern on what he saw as ageist attitudes and behaviors among the largely immigrant staff at Wetherby Place. In his untaped interview, he described embarrassing bathroom encounters with staff before he was able to manage his toileting needs independently and complained that staff members smiled at residents for no reason, called his peers "cute," played childlike games with balls, and cajoled resistant older adults by saying, "Do this for me." He believed these actions turned residents into children and the staff into parent-like supervisors. Mildred Ashman, also residing at Wetherby Place, disagreed with Mr. Levenson about the staff, saying, "*I appreciate what they do—which I really do and think that's one reason they're so good to me. I really do appreciate what they do. It's not an easy job—it's not a high paying job. You know they're not doing it all for the money.*" Mr. Braskey, a third resident of Wetherby Place, claimed that a dedicated staff member, "*saved my life because I gave up. And she brought my—gained my interest back,*" after he lost his wife and suffered a debilitating stroke, both of which left him deeply depressed.

Another example of variation relating to choice and autonomy concerned which choices mattered. For example, Mr. Cohen enjoyed many aspects of Wetherby Place, appreciating the privacy of his room and bathroom, as well as the staff's attention and sense of humor. When asked about what made Wetherby a quality AL, his reply focused on food, "*for every meal they give us a choice of two menus. Plus if we don't like either of the two, we can order something else, that's not one of the two. One thing I like about it is—the choice.*" For others, choice was about how to spend their time, or where to spend it. Hobbies, trips outside the AL, phoning friends, resting, reading, or helping others filled the days for many, as will become clearer in later chapters.

As we will show in greater detail in subsequent chapters, the mixture of elements identified as priorities for quality was extensive. Peter Granier admired the Greenbriar as a quality place for its ambiance, food, and leadership. "*Well, it's a beautiful place—and every room that I've been in—I've been in several rooms, don't get me wrong—and they all seem nice. They're clean and I liked that dining room as soon as I walked into it, and the food has always been good. When I first came here,* [current executive director] *wasn't here yet, but she made a big difference in this place."* Mr. Dugan, who initially said a good day depended on whether his television was working, complained mostly about the location of the Greenbriar. *"Well, it's the boondocks.... To me, that's the whole thing. I mean you can't go around and walk around. I mean, you can't go outside there and walk a ways. Where I was in [old neighborhood], I could walk to the stores, I could walk to the mall, I could walk to a restaurant—a lot of things.... You're isolated here, like you say. I mean all you got is this little shopping center across the road and you don't dare cross the road with the traffic here...."*

These examples and many more suggested that quality in AL is not about a single or even a few key elements that are widely shared. Instead, there is a long list of possible items that make a difference for individual residents, with many potential combinations. And, while broad themes, like food, staff, or the physical environment, may resonate with many individuals, the particular elements within these themes vary across individuals in shaping a sense of quality (e.g., is liking the physical environment really about the public spaces, where the AL is located, or how much space/storage there is in the rooms). In short, the basis of any specific resident's view of AL quality rests upon a specific set of criteria for that person. Evaluating quality becomes increasingly complex when we try to identify shared priorities across groups, such as staff or family members.

This very complexity in how quality is evaluated challenges us to find ways to develop, sustain, and evaluate quality in AL settings. When large numbers of participants in the daily life of AL hold varied quality priorities, no "one size fits all" approach can possibly achieve universally high quality rankings, as was seen among the three women from Murray Ridge profiled earlier in this chapter. While this challenge seems substantial, a surprising number of residents expressed overall positive views of the ALs where they lived, which they sometimes also called "home."

Question 3: Quality Compared to What?

Everyone entering AL has prior exposures that serve to frame their lives in this new environment—lived experiences that frame expectations.

At a minimum, one's home before coming into AL serves as a potential reference point. While some of those we interviewed told us they had little or no experience with long-term care prior to their own move to AL, others had relatives', friends' or their own experiences in a prior care setting that also served as a frame of reference in which to compare and evaluate where they now lived.

Where I Used to Live   Many people we interviewed realized that it was no longer feasible for them to live in their old homes or apartments, and several mentioned not missing tasks like cooking, cleaning, or climbing stairs. Nonetheless, feelings about long-time homes ran deep, and many people compared both physical and psychological dimensions of that home with their current life in AL.

Ms. Salguiero had previously lived in a high-rise apartment for seniors in another part of town prior to moving to St. Brigid's. *"I'm not happy. All my happiness is going. I had everything I want,"* she said, referring to all the wonderful things in her apartment and the social life she led there. In that apartment, she could look out the large picture window of her sixth-floor apartment, watching the moon and the airplanes above and the cars below. Now, she said with much sadness, *"I don't see any airplanes, I don't see any moon, Oh!"*

Jill Kates from Wetherby Place longed for her former life and home. *"[F]or a while there I had my own place—with my grandson. I had . . . what they call the mother-in-law apartment. And I was happy there. I mean, I didn't need anybody around me. At least I could see my little great grandchildren. Every day I would watch them at the swimming pool— watch them on the tennis court, you know. I was enjoying life. That was all taken away—and it kind of bothers me. I've got to get over it. It's hard, it's very hard."* Her friend, a physician, advised her daughter to move Ms. Kates into AL. For her part, Ms. Kates said, given an opportunity, *"I'm going to really give it to him"* [her physician friend] for making that recommendation. Ms. Powell of St. Brigid AL also missed the independence she enjoyed in her apartment. *"You're more independent. Like here, you're not independent because you can't do what you want for yourself. They have activities here but, like I said, in the apartment— you could go when you want and come when you want. You didn't have to say—I'm going so and so—and I'll be back in that time . . . No, I like it in an apartment better."*

Prior to moving to the Greenbriar, Ms. Brubaker lived in a unique house, built to provide wheelchair access for her late husband, which enabled her to remain at home as her own health declined and she came, eventually, to use a wheelchair herself. After managing at home for years, eventually suffering for months with an unreliable home health aide, she chose to move to AL. But clearly that special house, and her long years of living there, served as her primary frame of reference for assessing life in the AL. When asked about the Greenbriar, Ms. Brubaker found evaluation difficult. *"I don't know, because I lived there for like 40 some years in my house and I guess I try to compare everything else with it."* In addition to practical comparisons, residents often held strong emotional bonds to home (Rubinstein, 1989). At Boxwood Gardens, Ms. Gentile summed this up by saying, *"Oh, no contest— living home is your home. You have a dear love of it. I don't have a dear love of* [this place]. *It's a facility that I need, and that's how it is. But my home was my joy."*

Where Residents Received Prior Care   For many of the residents interviewed, the current AL was not the first stop for care, with many having prior rehabilitation or AL stays. These provided another point of comparison for current daily life in AL. William Gray, for example, had a poor prior AL experience and liked Winter Hills by comparison. He said, *"... it wasn't a very good place. To me it was like living in jail. This little old room—the meals weren't good, I'm telling you like it is—weren't too good. Like crackers and milk or something like that every day for meals."* Ms. Morris said of her prior nursing home stay before moving to Boxwood Gardens, *"it was like hell."* Mr. Braun found the Winter Hills staff more responsive than those who had cared for him during his rehabilitation stay and praised their call system that avoided long waits he'd faced in the prior setting. In contrast, Mr. Levenson, who moved to Wetherby Place after a stay at a university teaching hospital, found many members of his AL's staff to have an "attitude" when compared with staff at the hospital and said that they *"can be nasty,"* which made daily interactions unpleasant for him.

Others, like Mr. Cohen, focused on elements of space and privacy. While he admitted that he received good medical care and "got better" in his prior rehabilitation care setting, when asked to compare it to Wetherby Place, he said:

Mr. Cohen: Compared to what we have here, I didn't like it. What we had in rehab—we had two in a room and we shared bathrooms, so we had four people using one bathroom.

Researcher: What did you expect this place [AL] to be like?

Mr. Cohen: [O]f all the places where I've been, in the hospital and rehab and here, I like this place best..... Because we almost have our place. We have a private room, a private bathroom, so I really like this place better than the hospital.

Where Close Others Received Care A number of those we interviewed had experienced nursing homes or AL when others, either family or friends, had stayed there. Mildred Ashman employed her life experience of nursing homes, visiting her two grandmothers and her mother, as her frame of reference for her current situation at Wetherby Place.

Researcher: How did those places compare to this place?

Ms. Ashman: They weren't as nice as this—and now that I look back, I see a lot of things that are much nicer here...Doesn't look much like a nursing home.

Researcher: What do you mean by that—what looks less like a nursing home?

Ms. Ashman: It's got the nice lobby here and you don't see people sitting around tied in their chairs....That was one thing I really looked for when I was placing my mother—not to have that.

Ms. Riggs also spoke of her sister's time in a nursing home that she and a church group visited regularly for a prayer service as informative prior to coming to Arcadia Springs. "*And I mean—most of them had a terrible odor and they don't treat you right, and you lay and lay [unattended].*" On advice of her doctor, she investigated AL instead of a nursing home when she needed care. Ms. Pollock of Boxwood Gardens noted how times had changed. "*Well, you know like when I was young—like once you got along in years, my grandma lived with us and my mother was in a nursing home because she had a bad stroke....But I think more and more...everyone works. Now they have to go to this...this kind of place is necessary, I guess.*"

Today's Alternatives   Beyond what they had seen or experienced before, many residents who were interviewed discussed alternatives to their current AL for care, including competitors or living with family members. Ms. Carson of Boxwood Gardens had considerable experience, since she had friends living in other settings and had considered several different places, each of which she ruled out for being too large, too depressing, too expensive, or in the wrong location. Having put down a deposit at a large Continuing Care Retirement Community (CCRC) in her area, she gradually became disenchanted. *"And I kept watching it grow—and grow—and grow, and [that's] fine if you're a good walker and all, but I'm not. And I like a small group of people. One hundred fifty is fine with me—and get to know them. And, as I say, I don't like high rises. I feel like a bird in a cage, sort of claustrophobic and I don't like being up high and away from the earth. And so, that became out of the question, and it became financially out of the question, also."* Others, including Martha St. John, thought about places other than her current residence at Boxwood Gardens, but worried about the high costs depleting finances. In several cases, resident interviews revealed cost as among the necessarily important factors in their choice of an AL setting.

A different example comes from Dr. Styles, a retired university professor at Greenbriar Assisted Living. Dr. Styles knew a number of his university colleagues who had chosen a large CCRC not far from the Greenbriar. Having visited friends there, he considered both settings when it was time to move, focusing on the social environment and his personal preferences. Describing the CCRC, Dr. Styles said, *"The people over there, the ones I know, they are, generally speaking, an educated lot.... I expect that their family income has been pretty good and they're used to having—to participating in cultural activities of one kind or another. I'm not sure that's the same here."* He summarized it by saying, *"But I think the cultural level here is different than it would be over at [the CCRC]."* Asked whether he felt comfortable in his choice of the Greenbriar, he said *"I'm comfortable with it, yeah. I've never been much of a social lion. When I hiked, I hiked alone. Very seldom with somebody else—even one other person, very seldom. Reading is a solitary sort of thing. Listening to music is a solitary thing. Watching television is a solitary thing; it's not a participating sort of thing. I've not been a joiner."* Dr. Styles added that he liked that the activities staff *invited* him to be involved but did not pressure people to participate; he added that he would encourage others to choose a place based on what fit best with their lifestyles. *"If I was talking to somebody who was accustomed to going out to parties, to cultural events, going down to the theatre, going down to the opera—you know, that kind of participation—this would not be the place. That would be* [the CCRC]."

In contrast, some residents had expected—or hoped—to live with kin, particularly adult children, instead of moving to AL. As an example, Ms. Rosenstein, despite residing at Wetherby Place for 4 years, said, *"I don't feel at home here at all...I hate it here. The nurses are very nice, everybody's nice but I still hate the fact that I'm in a home."* Despite being unable to walk following a stroke, her desire to live elsewhere persisted. *"I would love to go to my daughter's house. She has a big home, 5 bedrooms...4 bathrooms... Of course I would need a nurse 24 hours."* Ms. Powell hoped she could leave St. Brigid and live with her sister, but then went on to describe the complicated family support system that enabled the sister, who'd had two strokes, to continue to live in her home, as well as the difficulty she would have with the stairs there. At least in St. Brigid, Ms. Powell said, she was *"treated with dignity and respect,"* unlike the old nursing homes.

In contrast, Ms. Larson said of the decision to move to the Greenbriar, *"...it was my own. I didn't want to go live with any of them. Most of them are boys anyway and it isn't the fact that they're boys, it's the fact that I really don't know their wives, not that well. I've met them and been with them and this and that—I don't know, it wouldn't be like being home."* Jean Thompson, discussed earlier in the chapter, mirrored others in recognizing the constraints of living with children or other kin. *"In a different age, people stayed home and take care of their loved ones—now I realize...there are so many women who have to have outside jobs. They aren't free to take care of their folks."* Wilma Harbaugh also said that it was her choice to move to Winter Hills, rather than to live with her children. Voicing this autonomy, she said, *"I know some people they hollered that their daughters put them in here. I said, 'Nobody put me here, I did it my own self, because I didn't want to live with them.' They just got married and I didn't want to be with them."*

A few residents also imagined that they might return to a home or apartment with paid help, feeling the loss of privacy or independence of life in AL. In some cases, the desire was to return to a native state or area where they would feel more "at home." However, many interviews with residents noted the high costs of personal care at home and concerns about safety or adequate support while living alone again. Others continued to wish their finances would permit them to relocate to some more expensive local care settings they had visited.

Question 4: Quality From Whose Perspective?

One of the study's central questions was how one's role in AL influences views of quality, both the elements chosen to form a framework for evaluation and the resulting quality "score." In their roles as residents, direct care staff, family members, or managers, these AL participants use very different frames of reference to "see" AL, resulting in varied views of quality. A recent study of end of life in AL found that staff members and family held very different views about those situations, which could lead to misunderstandings (Rich, Williams, & Zimmerman, 2010). Although we're focusing on views of residents here, the quality meanings of other key AL participants, including staff and family members, will appear more prominently in certain chapters. We provide a brief overview of the diversity of views across groups in this section.

As discussed earlier, whether a particular setting is deemed to be of good quality depends on what elements enter into the evaluation process—in short, what matters most from that person's perspective. As we interviewed members of each of these four groups, asking them similar questions about quality for themselves, their relative, or "residents" as a group, we saw the differing frames of reference emerging, revealing different priorities on what made life good for older adults living in AL. Interviews with staff and managers added some concepts that were not brought to light in interviewing residents. Direct care staff, for example, thought that the quality of the relationships between themselves and their managers/bosses was important to residents' quality, while this aspect was not noticed by residents. Similarly, in the card sorting activity mentioned earlier, family members ranked several items differently than did residents. More family members rated having uninterrupted sleep at night as highly important and having attractive grounds around the AL as unimportant to their relatives in AL, contrasting markedly with the residents' actual rankings on these items.

A second reason to expect differences in groups' perspectives on quality arises from differences in the reasons they might have for assessing quality. For providers and staff, for example, state regulations, company policies, and concerns about their competition may encourage a very different kind of quality review process than that undertaken by a daughter trying to decide whether to move or keep her mother in a given AL setting. The first group necessarily focuses on meeting regulatory priorities regarding medications, safety, physical plant, food service, staffing, and so on—items that may be subject to inspection or audit. It is this "provider perspective," focusing on physical (e.g., room types/sizes), staffing, services, and fiscal elements of AL operation, that has dominated much of the evaluation of "quality" in AL to date. These influences are distinct from the motivations to evaluate quality among older adults experiencing daily life among their peers in the setting, whose experiences are heavily shaped by daily encounters with people, routines, and requirements of living with others (see Chapter 2 for further discussion of collective living). Comparisons from the card sort results show some similarities and some differences across groups. For example, residents as a group placed lower priority in comparison to family and staff on having the AL building locked at night, the variety of activities available, having other residents of similar health status to themselves, how well managers respond to their requests, and having a staff that knows individual likes and dislikes. These items were clearly more important in the perspectives of family and staff groups than they were for older adults living in AL.

Key Elements in Understanding Residents' Perspectives on Quality

Based on our research and lengthy discussions, there are several key elements to better understand quality from the perspective of residents. **First, quality does not exist in the abstract**. Each of the older adults residing in an AL setting comes to that experience with a lifetime of housing, familial, social class, and other frames of reference to apply to the AL setting. In turn, each of the settings we studied had its own particular culture, leadership style, profile of residents and staff (in terms of background, class, health, culture, etc.) who shared a specific physical environment, community, and goals. In short, each place was distinctive and offered its own "brand" of AL, distinct from competitors in many ways that might be viewed as positive or negative. Carole Issacs, for example, emphasized that her lifelong orientations persisted in AL; she considered no one setting suitable for everyone.

> **Ms. Issacs:** *I really don't mix in too much. Now this one lady—oh, she's a dear lady and I love her, and she likes me, we get along real good. But she talks—she sits down the hall all the time in her wheelchair and talks, talks, talks and she likes it. But I'm by myself—but I'm happier that way.*
>
> **Researcher:** You're happier....?
>
> **Ms. Issacs:** *I'm not a mixer. I wasn't even when I was at home. I always enjoyed getting back to my home. Being to myself.*

In fact, the attention by each provider to creating a specific market niche for their AL was a growing consideration while our study was underway. ALs were trying to identify how they were distinct, special, or better in comparison to their proximate competitors, in order to attempt to capture consumer attention. These setting profiles and cultures are likely to be a part of what attracts particular individuals to choose one AL over another.

Second, quality is not static but rather is an ongoing process of review. Quality is created, with daily opportunities for revision during the everyday encounters and events that constitute life in AL. Through the work of staff, the choices of management, the daily actions of delivering services, and social dynamics among residents, family, and others, opportunities to define and reconsider quality are constantly emerging for all of the participants in the setting, particularly those who are there constantly—the residents. Quality is not achieved through a good state inspection or stellar customer satisfaction survey, becoming a fixed trait of a setting; instead it is necessarily in constant flux. This flux is driven by the arrival and departure of residents, staff, and leaders; as needs or capabilities shift for those living and working there; or as organizational changes, such as new ownership, an altered competitive environment or regulatory changes occur through time. Maintaining quality, regardless of whose frame of reference is used to establish it, remains an ongoing challenge in AL; its achievement is subject to constant review by those both providing and using its services. Central to our results is the conclusion that quality evaluations are likely not the same for all participants, whether we compare residents in the same AL setting, or look across settings. Although there are some common elements, what matters most in determining quality varies from person to person.

Third, each AL is more than a building with a staff which provides services, so consideration of quality must extend beyond these domains. ALs are places where some people work, others visit, regulators visit to ensure that minimum standards are met, and where people live and interact with an array of others on a daily basis (Carder & Hernandez, 2004). While they are businesses, they also are multiyear residences for people whose daily lives, friendships, hobbies, and interests become part of that community's flavor; for some it is their final home. For example, Mr. Braun of Winter Hills took pride and felt connected to his AL through displays of his wood crafting work in public areas of the building. Even AL settings that are part of chains, ostensibly sharing an overall philosophy of service and management culture, develop their own unique flavors based on their geographic location, the profile of clients they attract, and the constellation of skills and personalities among the staff employed there.

Fourth, one's role in the AL setting creates a frame of reference that is critical to identifying the essence of AL quality. As Jean Thompson noted earlier in this chapter, what she thought was important changed when she became a resident, rather than a family member visiting someone living in AL. The reality of spending most of your days and nights within the walls of AL is quite distinct from working daily shifts or visiting for limited periods of time. Similarly, the focus of attention by a member of the housekeeping staff is likely to differ from that of someone preparing meals or running activities, since what each of them "sees" as the heart of the AL's work differs. Administrators, too, see a differently inflected view than family members, having responsibility toward owners and regulators not shared by other groups. So when quality is discussed, taking into account the priorities of the person responding and how that person sees AL, it is not surprising that different people mean different things when they talk about quality.

How Do Residents Rate Quality in AL?

Although quality improvement initiatives focus on what's lacking, our interviews with residents encouraged them to focus on both positive and negative aspects of daily life and care within AL. Residents' views included some highly positive ratings of the ALs in which they resided, some that focused primarily on the negatives and other, more nuanced views that showed both benefits and constraints of daily life in AL. For example, two men living at Winter Hills, one of the more upscale settings in our study, independently mentioned that living there was like "heaven" for them. As you might expect, both identified numerous positive aspects of their lives there, focusing on getting along with people, the caring attitudes of staff, and other intangibles. Another resident, Ms. Dunn, whose main critique of Murray Ridge was wishing *"you could smoke in your room . . . [e]specially on rainy days,"* was, nonetheless, mostly positive about her life in AL. *"Keeping a bunch of old ladies happy—that's not easy, you know. But they do a damn good job."*

Ms. Gentile focused on the direct care staff at Boxwood Gardens, saying *"They're very caring, very patient. They're very kind, no matter what you need. They'll find an answer for you."* Aside from the necessities, such as cleaning the bathroom and changing her bed linens, she added, *"I find them very competent, I bless them every day, because they are caregivers. I'm a care taker and they are caregivers and they do a fantastic job."* Sharing similar views was Ms. Hite, whose interview emphasized St. Brigid's caring and pastoral focus. *"Like I say, they're all very caring . . . they go right out to try to help you and comfort you."* While she complained that her room was cold in winter and that the menu was adding to her waistline, still gave St. Brigid a "98%" for a grade.

Close to the end of our interviews with all groups, we asked participants to give the AL where they lived, worked, or visited a grade and to explain their reasons for selecting it. Some provided a numeric score, others a letter grade; all were converted to letter grades. First, residents gave the most "A-level" grades (53.7% between A+ and A−), followed by staff and administrators (40%) and family members, where 35.3% gave an A-level grade. Few of the ALs in the study were rated as poor or failing, with only one resident and one staff member giving such low evaluations. We might expect that family members, acting in their roles as advocates, were vigilant for problems, and consequently more likely to be critical. Both residents and staff members, however, may need to reconcile themselves to the limitations of their current living or work environment and take an approach that focuses on the positive aspects. Research on older adults also suggests that the brain's focus shifts toward positive information (George, 2010), perhaps enabling more residents to look on the bright side of what is, in many cases, not their preferred place to live.

A Note on the Use of Terminology

In this book, we sometimes refer to interviewees or groups by collective terms, such as staff, family, or residents. These terms, most particularly "resident," have been critiqued as shrinking individuals' complex identities, ignoring the distinctiveness of and value found in the individuals comprising these groups. For example, some claim that using the collective term "residents" reduces accomplishments, interests, histories, and personalities down to a narrow focus on current diagnoses and care needs. In our research, we have heard more stigmatizing generalities used, such as a staff member identifying one resident as "nursing home material" or another as "the two-person lift." Terminology was even mentioned by some of those we interviewed, including Mr. Grier, who said, *"This is a lovely place. As I told you before, we're not patients here, we are residents. And they treat you as a resident. Everybody here—You watch and see . . . [Staff is] orientated [sic] that we are not patients in this place here, we are residents."*

We appreciate the dilemma of employing these terms to identify our groups; our use of them is only linguistic shorthand which fully recognizes that there is considerable diversity within each group (Thomas, 2004). As will become clear, our work expands, rather than limits individuals' identities in AL to include their preferences, histories, and unique trajectories through life, as they reflect upon assessments of quality.

Profile of Coming Chapters

The focus of this initial chapter has been on the lack of a delimited and shared view of what constitutes quality in AL among residents.

Doubtless this reflects variations in individual backgrounds, expectations, and current frames of comparison. It also reflects the mixed and evolving role of AL—whether it is in fact a health care setting or a setting providing limited, non-medical support whose role is primarily social. This includes the core debate as to whether we're discussing quality of life or quality of care.

In coming chapters, we'll broaden the discussion of quality in several ways. First, in Chapter 2 we'll examine aspects of living in a collective setting (what we call a "soft institution") that entail major adaptations of daily life that are very different from most adults' prior living experiences in their own homes. Chapters 3 and 4 untangle the complexities of meaning that underlie two seemingly simple topics that are often discussed in connection with quality: staff and food. In both of these chapters, we examine how simply asking questions like "How is the food?" or "How well does the staff meet your needs?" is inadequate to understand the complexity of the culture of caring or the multifaceted reactions to food/dining/nutrition. Chapter 5 explores how autonomy and choice are enabled or thwarted in AL in light of the need for safety, as well as the pressures this places upon participants in AL life to negotiate solutions on a daily basis that sometimes undermine residents' assessment of quality. Chapter 6 explores the impact of regulation, including both state regulations and corporate policies, on how daily life unfolds for residents. In particular, there are interpretations of regulations on the ground, including some that attempt to individualize outcomes but still protect the institutions from risk or non-compliance. How residents perceive—or fail to see—the impact of regulation on the quality of their daily lives is also addressed. Chapter 7 examines the very fluid nature of quality over time, since both people residing in AL and the settings themselves change over time. The notion of quality balance between person and place and the potential for "everyday assessment" of quality among residents mean that our snapshot surveys really are only valid at one point in time. Finally, Chapter 8 provides recommendations for how to incorporate resident views when making daily or long-term choices and decisions within AL.

REFERENCES

Ball, M. M., Perkins, M. M., Whittington, F. J., Connell, B. R., Hollingsworth, C., King, S. V., Elrod, C. L., & Combs, B. L. (2004). Managing decline in assisted living: The key to aging in place. *Journal of Gerontology: Social Sciences, 59*(4), 202–212.

Carder, P. C., & Hernandez, M. (2004). Consumer discourse in assisted living. *Journal of Gerontology: Social Sciences, 59B*(2), S58–S67.

Eckert, J. K. et al. (2009). *Inside assisted living.* Baltimore, MD: Johns Hopkins University Press.

George, L. K. (2010). Still happy after all these years: Research frontiers on subjective well-being in later life. *Journal of Gerontology: Social Sciences, 65*(3), 331–339.

Hawes, C., Rose, M., & Phillips, C. D. (1999). *A national study of assisted living for the frail elderly: Results of a national survey of facilities.* Beechwood, OH: Myers Research Institute, Menorah Park Center for the Aging.

Lawton, M. P., & Nahemow, L. (1975). In M. P. Lawton (Eds.), *Psychology of adult development and aging* (pp. 619–674). Washington, DC: American Psychological Association.

Mollica, R., Sims-Kastelein, K., & O'Keefe, J. (2007). *Residential care and assisted living compendium: 2007.* Available at http://aspe.hhs.gov/daltcp/reports/2007/07alcom.htm

Rich, S. E., Williams, C. S., & Zimmerman, S. (2010). Concordance of family and staff member reports about end of life in assisted living and nursing homes. *The Gerontologist, 50*(1), 112–120.

Rubinstein, R. L. (1989). The home environments of older people: A description of the psychological processes linking person to place. *Journal of Gerontology: Social Sciences, 44,* S45–S53.

Thomas, W. H. (2004). *What are old people for? How elders will save the world.* Acton, MA: VanderWyk & Burnham.

Wilson, K. B. (1990). Assisted living: The merger of housing and long-term care. *Long Term Care Advances, 1,* 1–8.

Zimmerman, S., Sloane, P. D., & Eckert, J. K. (2001). *Assisted living: Needs, practices and policies in residential care for the elderly.* Baltimore, MD: Johns Hopkins University Press.

Zimmerman, S. I., Gruber-Baldini, A., Sloan, P., Eckert, J. K., Hebel, J. R., & Morgan, L. A. (2003). Assisted living and nursing homes: Apples and oranges? *The Gerontologist, 43*(Spec. No. 2), 107–117.

2
The Everyday Experience of Quality in a "Soft Institution"

ORIENTING POINTS
- Moving to assisted living alters daily life and personal routines.
- Receiving assistance in an assisted living setting requires some sacrifice in regard to independence and privacy.
- Group living is geared to the majority's cognitive and physical capacities and interests.
- Residents learn to balance their expectations of life in assisted living with the realities found in the setting.

DINING AT THE GREENBRIAR

The dining room at the Greenbriar is an elegant and friendly place. A wall of windows looks out over the enclosed courtyard, and the tables are dressed daily with fresh flowers, colorful linen in yellow and green, glass goblets, and heavy stainless flatware. At any given meal, the wait-staff compliment or tease residents; the cook, a South Asian immigrant, converses with residents about their day and the menu she prepares; and the dietary head, when not overwhelmed with culinary logistics or suffering from migraine, mingles among the tables with friendly conversation. Few people complain about the food at the Greenbriar...and no one more often than Mr. Dugan.

Mr. Dugan, when he comes to a meal, shares a table with two other men. As in most assisted living (AL) settings, dining room tables are assigned by staff, ostensibly according to personalities and interests. Dr. Styles, Mr. Granier, and Mr. Dugan occupied other places in the dining room until a death of one resident and the transfer of another's wife into an Alzheimer's unit resulted in their placement together.

Despite similarities of gender, age, and socioeconomic status, they are a varied group; the table, in fact, reflects three distinct dyads within this triumvirate.

Mr. Dugan, a retired accountant, moved into the Greenbriar at the instigation of his daughters. He was a resident of a mid-Atlantic state, living on his own; an accident propelled him into the hospital and then to a rehabilitation facility. His family, in concert with his physician, decided he could no longer live alone, and so one of his daughters agreed to move him out of state and into an AL near her home. Mr. Dugan has never liked the Greenbriar, but probably would not like any institutional place. He wants an apartment by himself in his old neighborhood and is willing to hire at-home caregivers to keep an eye on him, if he could only move back. His health has failed several times. He had a heart attack and was also hospitalized from injuries related to falling.

Although it doesn't feel like home, nonetheless Mr. Dugan's small room has become a social hub for staff. "*Let them come in,*" he told the researcher, "*let them rest a little bit. Because I don't think they're paid enough to begin with. I think they get—I don't know what they get paid, but it's low.*" Making many of his meals (e.g., sandwiches) in his apartment and wanting to be the perfect host, he keeps two refrigerators full of food and drink to suit everyone's appetite: cold cuts, muffins, canned soft drinks, gallons of ice cream, and bottled coffee drinks. When his supplies are low, his daughter trucks in a wheeled cart, piled with cartons and bags, and then stores the items as best she can, out of sight. Mr. Dugan spends much of his day reading the newspaper, watching television, and going out with his good friend and table-mate, Mr. Granier.

Long retired from the postal service, Mr. Granier moved into Greenbriar willingly after a major fall and long period of rehabilitation in another care setting. His one requirement, he told his sons, was that the AL chosen had to be near his old neighborhood. "*I wanted a place close to home and a place where I knew the area, because I drive. And I wanted to be able to drive around where I knew.*" Located on a busy thoroughfare, the Greenbriar was familiar to Mr. Granier, but "*I never had an idea what this place was, and I drove past here hundreds of times. When I had to [find a place]—I found out what it was.*" Mr. Granier had been through a 4-month recuperation period in

Greenbriar, entering in a wheelchair, transferring to a cane, and eventually walking unencumbered as his health improved. Mr. Granier befriended Mr. Dugan, realizing that he was unhappy. The two went frequently to the American Legion and VFW (Veterans of Foreign Wars) halls for meals and "to have a couple drinks." Their trips also included visits to the local barber for haircuts, which was much appreciated by Mr. Dugan's daughter. Mr. Granier attended his local parish church and undertook minimal shopping, buying food items the Greenbriar didn't offer. *"I eat a lot of fruit—yeah—I go out to [grocery shop] right up the road here and get cherries, peaches, pears, and that kind of stuff."* In the dining room, he said, *"I moved from one table to another,"* and eventually he found himself with Dr. Styles and Mr. Dugan as tablemates.

Dr. Styles is a professor emeritus of physical science, with a strong interest in history. In retirement, he suffered several major ailments, the last requiring time in rehabilitation. He realized that he could no longer live alone, and when, according to Dr. Styles, *"I was wearing out my welcome at [the rehab]; I looked at two places."* In the end, he decided on Greenbriar, because his first choice was at full capacity when he was ready to relocate. Dr. Styles moved in with minimal possessions— the activities director found him a recliner when a deceased resident's family was heading to the dumpster with one. His suite's furniture was limited, because he kept his apartment intact and had plans to eventually move to his first choice AL when space became available. Dr. Styles had been a loner for years, long divorced, with what he called a *"dysfunctional family."* Despite his solitary lifestyle, he adjusted quite well to collective living in AL, running a *"movie night"* on his own in the third floor lounge, with popcorn for residents. Beside this activity, Dr. Styles retained his cargo van, making periodic trips to his apartment, meeting for lunch with university colleagues, and shopping at the local supermarket. *"I'm driving on roads that I know, and I can make all right turns and, you know, I just know the way. I'm comfortable with it."* He also appreciated the Greenbriar's accessibility to the city bus system, which he frequently used for physicians' appointments and to shop.

The table is a trio of dyads. Mr. Dugan, despite clearly disliking his living situation (*"I'm not happy here—period. I've never been happy here."*) is an affable and amiable sort who gets along well with both of his tablemates. *"I have a table with my friends,"* he shared with the researcher, *"two guys—two other guys with me. It's nice."* Dr. Styles, on the other hand, is well aware that relationships at his table are mixed. *"I sit at a table . . . [where] there are three men, one of whom I don't really like at all. Another one . . . follows this first one around. . . . We get along fine. That one guy, I don't hardly talk with him. [pause] He's super critical of how I eat, what I eat, what I wear for clothes, all that kind of thing."* Mr. Granier did, in fact, call Dr. Styles a *"baby,"* and recounts that he "eats poorly," implying poor manners, especially for one so educated. But the tension may be more the result of perceived elitism on Mr. Granier's part, because he confides that the *"professor preaches"* to them at the table. He reflected in his interview that he would much prefer to dine *"at a table for two,"* if his wife were still alive.

Notwithstanding some friction between these men, they share important similarities: high degrees of independence, intact cognition, the ability to leave the AL at will, and minimal health issues for men of their ages, all atypical characteristics for this (and most) ALs. Despite dissimilar educational levels and job histories, and some political differences, the men get along. They talk during shared meals and, importantly, no one has asked for a change of table. But the challenges they face in negotiating these regularly shared dining experiences are ones they would not encounter at all outside the collective living environment of AL. If it were not for moving into the institutional setting, they would be at their respective homes, each eating alone.

Residents live collectively in an AL, and the dining room reflects that shared quality. Everyone eats together at set times in one space. ALs have rules, with many setting-specific, including: assigned seating; no changing seats without permission; proper dress and table manners; food carryout limitations, even for minimal snacks; no unruly behavior; food choices mandated by the chef, corporate office, or state-based nutritional oversight requirements; and assistive devices left at the door. Staff members circulate through the room or congregate in a corner, talking with each other, sometimes in loud voices, or speaking languages residents can't understand. Just as residents break the rules, slipping a slice of cake or a piece of fruit into their walker totes to eat later, staff do as well, resorting to using their first language when supervisors are absent, in defiance of the rules requiring everybody to speak English. As a microcosm of AL, the dining room represents institutional living.

INSTITUTIONAL LIFE IN AN ASSISTED LIVING

An institution is vaguely defined as an organization focused on a specific purpose. A definition more tailored to our study refers to AL institutions as "organizations providing residential care for people with special needs" (McKean, 2005). As in other types of "institutions" providing housing and care for older adults, the special needs of residents in AL revolve around medication administration, assistance with everyday living (bathing, laundry, meal preparation), and general oversight, especially for those people with dementia. There is an unavoidable bureaucratic quality about institutions. For AL, this trait is manifested through a set of formal and informal rules, with people in care staff and managerial positions making decisions enabling the setting to operate as smoothly and effectively as possible, given the circumstances and competency of individuals at any point in time. Rather than being a collective of people who live together by choice and with consensus, the AL is ruled by a body of officials who mandate tasks and responsibilities for everyone, staff and residents alike. This internal, hierarchical administrative system, despite being bounded by state and local regulations (see Chapter 6), provides a routinely efficient way of meeting most of the diverse and divergent needs of residents. A turnover in administration may have limited impact on the individuals living and working there because, as in a true bureaucracy, individuals are secondary to positions filled and rules executed (see Chapter 7).

Long-term care residences are akin to what sociologist Erving Goffman calls "total institutions" (Goffman, 1961). Although Goffman focused on more constraining institutional settings, such as prisons, mental institutions, and monasteries, the parameters of a physically separated, confining, regimented, staff-oriented, and bureaucratically organized entity fits several aspects of the AL sector, although the degree of fit to specific ALs varies. As he notes in his 1961 work *Asylums*, these institutions structure life around the principles of bureaucratic control. Although residents are dominated by staff, following Goffman's model, there emerge in the total institution processes of adaptation and resistance, resulting in the creation of an internal culture or "underlife." In our study, the ethnographic team examined the "underlife" of seven AL settings to discern the cultural processes and their meanings for quality in these institutional environments, as determined by residents.

What makes an AL an institution? The first element is the physical environment. Essentially, residents do everything in one physical location: eat, sleep, and interact with co-residents, who may or may not be their friends. There are public and private areas, lounges, and a wellness office, interspersed with residents' rooms. Boundaries exist, from locked doors to definitive perimeters encircling the settings. Goffman calls this "inmate culture," and some residents in AL jokingly refer to themselves as "inmates." Second, regulations abound, with staff concerns predominating in the interest of efficiency under conditions of perpetually tight funding. Third, there are relations of power that can and do appear between those residing in AL and those providing care and management of the setting. Although this shadow of domination sometimes fosters feelings of powerlessness, as expressed among residents, there are also examples of resistance as part of the "underlife" of AL, where residents modify what strongly annoys them or impinges too strenuously on their lives.

Our research team came to refer to AL as a "soft" institution, because our observations were not a perfect match with the extremes discussed by Goffman. For example, some people willingly move in or move out. They can come and go freely (within some boundaries) and generally are not penalized when they disobey rules like neglecting to sign out. There is also much understated flexibility in the rules (some residents keep coffee pots in their rooms, despite the fire hazard) and some negotiation of monthly fees. Residents hold some decision-making authority, however elementary, as evidenced by participation in Resident Councils, Food Committees, and family meetings. "Soft" essentially means that nothing is quite as hard and fast as in the "total institutions" discussed by Goffman and others, because AL is not as physically or socially confining and allows flexibility in its expression of group life and application of rules. The system is pliable both to better meet residents' "consumer-oriented" demands and, by doing so, to retain census. Although few would refer to an institution as warm and fuzzy, some AL settings—or select employees within them—demonstrate an impressive degree of caring and compassion, as discussed in Chapter 3. Each AL presents some form of an institution, but the degree of softness varies from one setting to another.

As an example of how softness appears, few living in Goffman's total institution would refer to it as home. Many living in long-term care residences do so, although the AL, most probably, has an institutional feel in terms of its physical setting and daily routines. One of the researchers writing in her field notebook described the "institutional feel" of Boxwood Gardens this way:

> Entering the building through a set of automatic doors, there are two seating areas walled off on the left and right by glass buttressing the main entrance. Visitors are greeted by a round table on which sits a floral decoration and daily newspapers. A configuration of furniture lies behind, making an effective use of a fireplace. Behind this wall is the dining room, and to the visitor's left are an elevator, stairwell and hallway housing public restrooms, and a corridor of rooms, including a nurse's station and hair salon. Forty-five degrees to the visitor's right is the concierge's desk, behind which are an open stairway and the beginning of the corridor to the private dining room and the dementia special care unit. To the visitor's right beyond the small seating area are offices, a TV lounge with fish tank, a craft/sun room, and the entrance to another corridor of AL rooms. Different sounds were coming from all the directions, capped by music piped in through speakers.

Although some AL settings are small houses on cul-de-sacs, the AL settings in this book are more like the structure presented in the previous description: buildings with automatic doors, public restrooms, wellness offices, and hair salons. The setting is "home," and residents remodel their rooms to reflect their individual senses of self, displaying possessions such as a collection of Hummel figurines, a collage of family photographs, or a bookcase chock full of novels, DVDs, and *Wall Street Journals*.

The AL "institution," in its "softness," does not physically resemble the hospital or prison. In fact, as one researcher noted,

> The upstairs corridor is pleasantly lit and sunny. Walls are of a pale yellow and ceiling fixtures line the corridor; the end of the corridor has two large windows, one facing directly out, and one at right angles. A table of live plants and two chairs sit in front of the windows.

And on another day a researcher wrote,

> Walking these halls is pleasant. The lighting is good, both from large cornered windows and [from] subtle overheads. Pale yellow

walls help. The artwork is floral ("biological-style" sketches of flowers) and reproductions from famous artists, e.g., Monet. Views from windows give a "neighborhood" feel: small street, townhouses, large field and trees, playground, backyards. Residents in the front and sides can look beyond the parking lots into the community.

There is a definite intent to deinstitutionalize the building, with some residents taking this on in their own suites. Ms. Pollock accommodated to downsizing her apartment by sleeping on the couch. She gave away her bed so her small room would look more "homey" and less cramped, preferring to reside in a "living" room rather than one room that shouted that it was a "bedroom."

The Impact of the Institution on the Culture of AL Daily Routines

Within the AL, the impact of the institution is felt every day, from the time a resident rises in the morning to when she retires at night. A resident who elects to go to meals must be up and dressed in daytime attire by the time breakfast is served. There are AL settings where residents have voted to come to the dining room in bathrobes and slippers, but this is rare; and in other studies we have conducted, this issue has come up for discussion periodically but never has been acted upon. Staff, however, appear accepting of this idea. In one interview, the researcher asked a care aide what she would not like if she were to live at St. Brigid. She replied:

> I'll tell you the truth, I don't like to get dressed before I have my breakfast and they're fully dressed sitting there eating breakfast, but I wouldn't want to go out in my nightgown in front of anybody. So, I don't know what [would] be the ability of someone just coming up to a little buffet in their robe and have their breakfast in their room, fully functional. Something like that I would like. Because not every morning do I want a big breakfast. And you know how you really just don't feel like getting dressed yet? You want to go back to sleep for a while. I don't want to be up at the crack of dawn. Now, when I'm older and need to go there, I may

get up at the crack of dawn, I don't know. But right now, I do not, and I get up to have a cup of coffee, make sure the world is still out there and then I go back to sleep sometimes. So I would like the meals just a little bit different. So that I could do something like that, you know? And I don't think that's terrible seeing someone walking a hallway with a robe and slippers on, that's their home.

In fact, residents do speak about disliking the morning routine:

I can't get up in the morning and rush. And I say, please don't rush me because I get up—I'm stiff and hurting, and I forgot to take my nitroglycerin patch off last night, and I woke up this morning with one of the worst headaches you ever had from that nitroglycerine. . . . I can't be rushed because . . . I can't breathe . . .

A resident who is independent can toast a muffin in his room, like Mr. Dugan does. Others must make their way to the community dining room to get their first cup of coffee, and if ground coffee has for some reason not been delivered to the kitchen, must wait until another day for a cup. Breakfasts—eggs, bacon, sausage, pancakes—are overwhelmingly the most popular and most appreciated, if not the most healthy, meal of the day, according to resident interviews. However, institutional issues appear here as well. All menus are dictated by the dietary manager or corporate office, with resident input sometimes elicited through food committee meetings, which may or may not result in meaningful change. It is not uncommon for residents to submit their favorite recipes for consideration, or to ask for a favorite of this cohort, liver and onions.

People who are not able to get themselves to the dining room—or any place in the AL—on their own are dependent on availability of staff members for transport, which can require a short, or long, wait. Self-mobility is encouraged, as it fosters exercise and lifts some pressure off staff. As part of daily routine, residents in many AL settings are required to sign out when they leave the premises, if only for a walk around the block. Most do; some forget. Ms. Ames refuses on principle because she is independent and where she goes is "no one else's business."

Institutionalization impacts both the major and the mundane. Laundry is placed in any drawer where a staff member finds space, rather than according to the resident's wishes. Ms. Carson at Boxwood Gardens hunted for nightclothes only to discover her gown buried underneath a pile of socks. Such actions are especially problematic for residents with health or vision difficulties, who are struggling to remain independent by memorizing locations of their possessions. Bathing schedules must be coordinated according to all residents' preferences and the schedule of care aides assigned to various corridors across shifts. A resident who was promised, by the marketing consultant, assistance with getting into her van when she signed her contract later discovered that such help was only forthcoming if a staff member was available and willingly agreed to this task. So although help and services are available, they are constrained by the requirements of the institution, including limits of staffing.

On a typical day, residents are inundated with a multitude of schedules. Let's return to dining as a key exemplar of these scheduling challenges. The AL is perhaps feeding 50–100 residents, with a rotating schedule of menus. Directors of Dietary Services have a sense of various things: what they can afford and what to buy seasonally; what can be efficiently prepared for large numbers of people, many of whom require specialized diets; and what meals are deemed appropriate to a restaurant-style dining room, where all of the residents want to eat at the same time. Mealtimes are also scheduled, with breakfast at 8, lunch at noon, and dinner at 5 p.m.—the most common meal times. Some settings are more flexible than others, and several supplied snacks at varied times during the day or offered food in a public location on a self-service basis. If a facility has a small dining room, it often needs to offer two seatings to accommodate everyone, and so some residents are "scheduled" to eat lunch at 11 a.m. and dinner at 4:30 p.m., followed by a second shift of residents taking lunch at noon and dinner at 5:30 p.m. When a resident inquired at a meeting if dinner could be served at 6:30 p.m., one dining services coordinator laughed in response. When the resident pressed, suggesting 6 p.m., the coordinator responded that he needed to get home. Despite the popularity of breakfast, in an AL requiring multiple seatings, it is the one meal where all residents wanting to eat fit into the dining room at the same time. Many residents like to sleep in, preparing something simple like cold cereal in their rooms instead of eating in the dining room. Not being able to have a hot breakfast when one wishes is another symptom of the institutional pressures under which ALs operate.

Residents also follow a schedule for laundry, housekeeping, bathing, medication, and activities. Field trips to the supermarket; excursions out to lunch; activities such as bingo, Pokeno, art club, exercise class, trivia, current events, movies, and live entertainment are typically scheduled on the same days and times each month. Conveniently, one can schedule doctors' visits and trips off the grounds or visits with friends in-house around an activity one likes or doesn't. Each resident gets an activity calendar to keep; a large one is generally mounted in a public place; and calendars are posted online for family members and researchers, who then knew where to find residents and what days to avoid. One resident commented:

> After breakfast I sit outside a while and I like the fresh air, and the
> sunshine. And intend to enjoy it, while we still have it. In the afternoon,
> they usually have some kind of activity after lunch. Music—they'll
> have a disc jockey, or a singer and then they have like socials out in the
> sunroom. They might have cake and ice cream or popcorn and Sprite, or
> smoothies—fruit smoothies—but there's always something going on in
> the afternoon.... [later in the interview] And on Wednesdays they have
> fingernail day, where the staff polishes your nails or files them and there's
> a little girl that comes in and does facials. I forget what company she's
> with—something like Avon or you know that type of thing. But she's very
> good. But that's Wednesdays—she'll come—you want your nails done
> today? And they have all kinds of polish and removers and clear coat, I
> only use clear coat, because I have a tendency to pick and I hate chipped
> fingernail polish, so I use clear. It doesn't show so bad, but they're very
> good. So everything that you really need is here and they're very good
> about it.

Schedules help staff do their job in a workplace where they are pressed for time. Some of the institutional feel of AL, from the perspective of some residents, arises from the way that staff are assigned to work. Ms. Carson describes what she finds at Boxwood Gardens.

> They keep rotating people around. I never know who's going to be coming
> into my room, or when. Now, I don't mind them coming into my room
> because if they do knock, they used to knock so hard that they jumped me
> out of bed . . . it doesn't really jump me out of bed, but my heart beats and

I get all upset, and my stomach gets upset. I can't stand that loud noise on my nerves. So I had a sign up for a long time, not to knock, but you know—to softly come in and say your name. After a while I took it down, because most of the time they don't take time to read the sign you've got up there. They're in a rush—and they rush in and rush out. I'm trying to talk to them, they're already out the door and halfway down the hall, and I'm talking to myself. They have no time. Now do we blame this on the nursing shortage?—I don't know.

Her daughter corroborates what she told us:

Boxwood Gardens wants to run on their schedule, they don't want to run on the resident's schedule. And I—you know what they tell you, they tout that it's your home now and you're to be treated like it is your home, but it's not. They have a schedule....and I understand that they need to have a schedule, because you do have to run things in that manner...but I think that they try to run their schedule rather than looking at the resident's schedule.

The Sociophysical Environment

When people move into an AL, especially if they are loners like Dr. Styles, the presence of people in the public spaces every day can be overwhelming. A total institution can resemble a little village, and the philosophy of AL advocates that residents socialize with one another, as noted by Darlene Hall in Chapter 1. They are encouraged to be out and about, conversing, criss-crossing in the halls to talk with one another, and gathering for a smoke outside in the rain. Despite this AL value that being social is a desired outcome for all, residents rarely visit in each other's rooms, except for wanderers with dementia who forget where they live. Staying mostly within one's room and rejecting participating in activities is (sometimes grudgingly) respected, however. Staff know that some people are most comfortable by themselves and have been loners for a number of years. Others appreciate and seek out company. Some residents do meet on their own in the fireplace lounge, "personalizing" public space, keeping each other posted on the latest family news, often with staff members joining in. Apartment doors are left open not only to embrace larger public spaces, but also for people to feel more connected to life beyond their individual rooms. Everyone seems to know everybody else's business, or think they do, and news travels fast among and between residents and staff in a tightly controlled environment. Ms. Brubaker at the Greenbriar, whose prior life hadn't been highly social, appreciates that she is able to choose how she uses her time.

> *I really don't have too much to complain about because if I get lonesome or anything, I can always go into these art class—and crafts. Or anywhere they're having exercise—it's something all day long. So any day that I feel like I want to go out there, I have the freedom to do it. If I feel like I just want to sit here and rest—or sleep—I have that freedom. That makes a good day for me.*

Personal privacy is one thing to consider in collective living. Environmental privacy is another. Doors, even locked ones, do not stop staff from entering living quarters unannounced to ask a question or check on a resident. In addition, care and housekeeping staff enter these supposedly private spaces while simultaneously knocking, announcing an activity, or a meal, or doing some housekeeping duty.

Locking doors is sometimes discouraged, primarily because care staff consider it a safety issue, as seen in the following dialogue between Georgia, a care aide at the Greenbriar, and our researcher:

> *Georgia:* You can't get to the room. We can't get into there. And sometimes they faint away or something happens.
>
> *Researcher:* So you don't have keys to the rooms?
>
> *Georgia:* No, we used to, but they take the keys, because some of the residents complaining that they have some things are stolen, so they don't give us key. Housekeeper they give key, but there are times they page them and the housekeeper not come. It's time grueling you know. That I don't like. Like here I'm working, and when I go to wake them up in the morning, most of my people are really on the third floor. So I just make sure they leave their door unlocked.

In the interview, Georgia goes on to reinforce that when she senses that something is amiss, she can have difficulty tracking down a key. Going down two floors to the main office to find one is valuable time lost if a resident is in distress.

On the other hand, Ms. Ames, whose independent nature we have already noted, has difficulty keeping her apartment locked. She can't trust the staff to lock her door. She tries to train the staff, but every time there is a staff change the new workers don't lock it. She doesn't understand why the management can't put this information in her record and then train new staff. She has a note taped to her door to remind staff that they need to turn off the lights and lock up. Even though she has posted this reminder on bright colorful pink paper, a lot of staff still ignore her wishes. Her requests to be taken off the list of routine nightly room checks have not been honored, and, consequently, she ends up having to get out of bed most nights and make her way to the door in the dark to check the lock after they visit.

> *I don't want to be disturbed at night. I don't—at this point I don't want them coming in and checking to find out if I'm asleep…they would come around every two hours, but if I'm sleeping I'm really enjoying the sleep—you have disturbed my sleep. So that's what my sign is about. I don't want them—but the thing is that every time the management changes or the staff changes then it happens over and over again and you find that you have to say it over and over again….I told them I'm putting up signs….they would come in and wake me up and I would say, please don't do this any more. And then I'm in the bed out of my wheelchair and then they leave…and they don't turn off the lights. They turn all the lights on—they don't turn off the lights and they don't lock the door. And when they came in they know they had to unlock the door, all right.*

Bodily privacy is a third concern for many living in a collective setting. Residents need assistance with tasks, exposing their bodies to inspection when showering or toileting. Residents are stripped down bare before the eyes of staff they barely know or may dislike. Gender issues sometime surface, with female residents uncomfortable with male aides, male residents appreciating the female caregivers' touch and conversation. AL settings will sometimes amend staff members' schedules to accommodate residents' requests for a staff member of a particular gender.

Another institutional aspect of AL is that noise permeates the setting day and night. Days are definitely more bustling because administrative staff are present in the facility and care staff numbers are greater. Besides, settings have the greatest number of activities in late morning and afternoon and so many residents are out and about. Noise is also influenced by daily schedules, because midday noise may be perceived differently from noises overnight. The AL structures its organization so that residents are ready for bed between 8 and 9 p.m., enabling the evening staff to finish by 10 p.m., before the arrival of the smaller staff employed for the 11 p.m. to 7 a.m. shift. Residents who are night owls are on their own to amuse themselves or meet any needs, given this limited staffing. Just because residents are put to bed does not mean that they sleep. Residents call out, often increasing in volume if their bells or call buttons are not answered; they get up, wander and chat, rarely in whispering voices; they moan in pain; their televisions may blare because the residents' hearing is impaired. Ms. Carson says,

> I didn't think I was going to have to help other people who are crying and screaming for help. They don't hear them down there at the desk. I had to get on my scooter several times. I went into someone's room once because he was yelling and carrying on...and then the other one...I tried to help him. I had to get on my scooter, out of bed, on my scooter, go down to the front and tell them at the desk, someone needs help down here in this room. They're calling "quick, help, help, quick"—I'm the only one that heard it.

ALs are busy places full of busy people, not collective settings with passive, laid-back individuals. Noises range from clicking shoes, shuffling feet, beepers and cell phones, to scraping chairs, intercoms, piped-in music and CD players, vacuum cleaners, casual and heated conversations, air conditioning units, and local traffic. Technology brings its own noise. A researcher writes in her fieldnotes that "Mr. Guarino," residing at Arcadia Springs, "has gotten so used to the noise [of his oxygen tank] that he doesn't even notice anymore." In her role as a researcher she was bothered by it, as well as by a wheeled cart "causing enough noise that I had to wait to proceed [to interview] until it passed."

Noise is not consistent across all settings or even within the same setting at varied times. At the Greenbriar, Ms. Larson says, "You never hear any noise in the hallways" whereas others, including staff, disagree. Ms. Cusick at Murray Ridge moved into a dementia unit because "she didn't like the noise and traffic that comes with living upstairs." In contrast, Mr. Burrell at Arcadia Springs feels that residents with dementia should be locked on another floor because of the noise they make. Some residents complain about noise; others ignore it, taking it in stride in an institutional setting; some actually find noise comforting; and others can't hear it at all! One sound that no one ignores is the siren. In her interview at Boxwood Gardens, Lindsay, Director of Marketing, tells us,

> …my desk is right near the window and I hear sirens and I'm like, "What's going on? Who is that?"—you know. Are they coming into the parking lot? I feel like residents, when they hear the sirens pull up, they all come to the lobby. They all want to know what's going on and I think some of it has to do with being nosy and you know wanting to know the scoop, and know what's going on before other people do. But I think some of it is—I think a lot of it is—that they are concerned it's one of their friends. They're concerned. We have some siblings that are here together and a couple of sisters that are here. It something that definitely puts people on edge, and sometimes the ambulance is here two or three times a day.

AL facilities are also workplaces and the staff call out to each other down corridors and across living areas throughout their shifts, day and night. Beth, a care aide at Arcadia Springs, finds that she needs to instruct coworkers that the AL is not only a place of employment but home to its residents.

> I mean, ones that are younger, they just don't get it yet that this is their [the residents'] home and we just work here. You know we work eight hours a day here, but they live here 24/7, you know? So this is their home and that's kind of a hard thing to get through to someone. And I can understand it, because you wouldn't think of it that way, but it is. And if you're working 11 to 7 shift, and you're out in the hallway giggling and laughing, being all loud, someone is trying to sleep in their room, in their home. How would you feel, you know?

Construction costs do not allow for soundproofing, so often these ongoing noises disturb those attempting to sleep. One thing is certain. Between AL's emphasis on sociability and the design of the physical environment, solitude is an impossible state in a collective setting.

Physical space is an issue when an AL allots a certain square footage per resident per monthly fee. Like people in all prime real estate, residents value size in their living spaces. Our researchers have observed that the smaller the room, the more crowded the space. Rather than living with minimal possessions and fully downsizing, residents fill closets until they overflow, store items in stacked bins around and under beds and chairs, and shove bags with belongings in every nook and cranny. Families will sometimes oblige by storing off-season clothing and most treasured mementos safely at their homes. Roommates negotiate shared areas, with the living rooms of two-person suites often resembling storage units rather than usable living spaces. What is apparent in a soft institution is that the social environment blends in with the physical setting, affecting cultural factors of daily life, including privacy and ambiance.

The Medical Dimension of the Soft Institution

The inability to easily manage one's life because of physical and/ or cognitive problems is the quintessential reason why people move into an AL. Residents do not move into an institution and relinquish some independence simply because the location or amenities are so inviting. It is an alternative form of housing, and few residents are like Dr. Styles—who rationally decided to come of his own volition. More residents come in "kicking and screaming," as one director told us. Resistance arises because they fear the loss of independence and because of the negatives of leaving the homes in which they have lived for the past 30–50 years. Older adults become AL residents because health and safety are huge concerns to their families and, often, to themselves.

In moving into the AL, the new resident and her family turn over some of the management of health care to those operating and providing AL services, a major task to put into the hands of a bureaucracy relatively unknown before she arrives. The AL takes over the daunting responsibility of making sure that the resident gets help with bathing, eats well, takes medications, remains upbeat, socializes with others, and has her nursing needs—like treatment of skin tears or application of eyedrops—attended to.

It must be remembered, however, that the AL is not a medical facility. Because they enter with health care needs, some residents assume that the AL operates like one. Some see the facility as a friendlier, more attractive, and cheaper alternative to a nursing home. These expectations, reflective of the medical model of care described in Chapter 1, can be unrealistic. Some residents feel that doctors should be on call, that physical therapy should be available in-house daily, or that their individual care aides should be licensed nursing staff. It is not uncommon to hear residents refer to each other as patients.

By and large, AL does an adequate job of meeting the residents' health care needs, especially in view of the fact that its goal is providing assistance, not specifically medical care. In its provision of health services, it is the institutional quality of the AL that is bothersome to some residents and their families. Ms. Hailey, the daughter of a resident, has observed, after talking to her mom, that "staff don't really talk to you. They're very...some of them are very cold and plain and—no smiling, no pleasantries. 'What do you want?' would be their response."

Scheduling, referenced earlier in this chapter, and medical assistance are the two most commonly noted institutional aspects of residential life. Ms. Kates, a resident at Wetherby Place, finds that these factors, in combination, present problems for her.

> ...they give you your pills every day—which to me in the State of Maryland is for the birds, because to me I'd rather have my pills right here in my medicine chest.... —so that's one thing I don't like—not allowed to have your pills. And when they give them to you—here I go again, but these people—I go for breakfast and at breakfast I take 7 pills, so I have my breakfast, I eat my breakfast then I sit there and I wait for my pills. Why they can't put those pills on the table for you? I can't understand....I eat and I sit there, and sit there, and sit there—...waiting for those stupid pills. They should put them on the table for you and when you come, sit down, take your pills, drink your water—they can watch you, but you should do it—that's how I feel. A person changes when they're sitting around waiting.

The institutional quality of AL is problematic for some more than others. Mr. Dugan realizes, "*I am here because I have to be here,*" accepting his fate for his daughters' sake. Dr. Styles recognizes the important function the institution serves and appreciates the fact that "*I can do what I want here.*" Mr. Granier has established himself within the institution, making friends with residents and management, and accepting life at the Greenbriar. "*I told everybody—I'm going to die here—if they let me.*"

Expressing Autonomy

As already expressed by Ms. Ames and Dr. Styles, finding ways to exercise independence is a crucial characteristic in the adjustment of many residents to AL, and, hence, later in the book, we devote an entire chapter to this topic. Long recognized by senior housing executives, independence has been a critical concept in the formation and current success of AL. How independence is expressed, however, is couched within the particular culture and environment of each soft institution.

It is rare for residents to come and go as easily as Dr. Styles and Mr. Granier. Driving his friend, an arrangement made between two cognitively able adults, required Mr. Granier to sign a risk agreement to take Mr. Dugan in his car. Independence is viewed within the parameters of what is allowed by the setting. At a tacit level, the facility boasts menu choices for its residents, and so residents may exert a sort of choice and control in everyday life by selecting a fruit plate over grilled steak. But choices are bounded by rules, and residents have choices only over certain things, things that AL, and the state regulations that govern it, decide. Food is definitely one key area where choice comes into play, most probably because residents are interested in food and encounter it three times a day. Besides, food is a relatively easy arena, in which facilities can offer choices. Dietary restrictions may, however, limit this choice. Most homes allow their residents with special dietary needs—for example, diabetics—to choose whatever foods they prefer, regardless of dietary recommendations. So if a diabetic opts to have pecan pie and rejects the sugar-free Jell-O, the resident's choice is honored. This reflects, characteristically for a soft institution, the fuzzy boundary between the medical model of care and the original AL philosophy of autonomy; the latter which honored choice for residents—including poor choices, such as the pie, which might have been made at the residents' previous homes.

AL settings make other rules about eating; residents sometimes adhere to them and, in other circumstances, break them. The director of the Greenbriar announced that food no longer was to be taken out of the dining room after meals. This annoyed several residents, including Ms. Jacobs.

> **Ms. Jacobs:**...*of course I'm very upset with this food business, that we can't bring the food back to your apartment. But it's like one or two students have a fight in the classroom and the whole class gets punished, that's just what it is, so...Because they have had to go around where some people brought the food back and didn't even put it in the fridge, and others put it in the fridge and let it get all moldy and everything. And they've had cockroaches. And [the executive director] said rats—I said, "Are sure you don't mean mice?" She said, "I mean rats."*
>
> **Researcher:** So nothing can come out of the dining room?
>
> **Ms. Jacobs:** *No, but I snuck my cake....[reading from the management directive] It says, "We discourage the removal and consumption of food from the dining room in common areas for these reasons." So I said to Jenny [another resident], they just discourage it, they didn't say I'd go to jail—I'm taking my cake...*

Ms. Jacobs's actions, defying this rule, are another way to express "softness" in an institutional setting, and her actions fall well within Goffman's model of resistance in the "underlife."

Degrees of autonomy are also reflective of the approach that is characteristic of each AL. Victoria, the director of Winter Hills equates rights with choice.

> To me, residents' rights—is being able—if you want to go to the dining room and sit there a half an hour early, it's your dining room. You should be able to do that. No one should tell you, "No, you can't go into the dining room," because it's considered common space and this is their home. Anything from that to what they want to dress and how they want to dress, you know. We [pause] we ask that everyone bathe at least once a week here for obvious reasons, but we're not going to tell someone, you know, they have to have a shower rather than a hot tub or spa. So to me residents' rights is respecting their choices.

Institutions do limit and modulate behavior. In order to have a smoothly running facility, they draw lines where independence ends and facility constraint begins.

Sexual activity may be reported to families, permission is asked of those with powers of attorney for residents to walk off the grounds, and families are contacted if residents refuse bed checks or baths.

Residents' autonomy is frequently overridden by the pressures on, and efficiency of, the institution. Although it is beneficial for residents to clothe themselves, it may be too time-consuming for the care aide to wait for each resident to select an outfit and painstakingly button her shirt. Within the institutional underlife, residents and staff quickly learn what expressions of choice to accept, to battle, or to manipulate. In an institution where everything is geared toward the "average" resident and the degree of efficiency mandated by management, Ms. Jacobs decided on subversion—to literally take the cake.

BALANCING QUALITY IN A SOFT INSTITUTION

The institution of the AL is a home to many older adults. But as a place where people both live and work, the AL necessarily takes on a bureaucratic nature. Elders move into a collective setting where, on a daily basis, they negotiate private and public spaces, share meals, adjust to a cacophony of sounds, conform to or undermine rules, move among people with varying physical and cognitive abilities, tolerate diversity, and adapt to surroundings that resemble a commercial environment more than a residential physical environment. Some residents adjust to this very well—others do not. Ms. Howe finds that Murray Ridge

> ...doesn't seem like an institution, you know. When it's breakfast time, we're down to eat our breakfast. If you're a little late nobody is going to holler at you—I love it here. I really do. I wish our mothers could have had something like this....I'm happy to be here and I thank the good Lord that I have a nice place to stay. I know that my family is glad that I'm happy and we all just look after one another....As you can see, I'm perfectly happy here. I am.

Some residents, like Ms. Carson, are on the other end of the continuum, however.

> What makes this a good life in assisted living? That depends, of course, on who you are. And we're all individuals. Institutional life is not really my style, but I do want to be around people. But I would say the purpose from the resident's viewpoint is to serve the needs of us as individuals, all of whom have serious medical conditions. Different—we're not all the same,

and we have different personalities. That's our standpoint. And I've talked to other patients here. They may not get as upset as I do, with everything inside of me ready to explode. . . . But they know and they tell me, and they say to me, the purpose of the corporation is to get as much money as they can to exploit the fact that we have a growing elderly population. And they are doing this at the expense of our health care, our personal care, house care—everything. They offer, at their convenience, a scheduled program. If you don't fit into that schedule, you're left out. And that is exactly what one of the patients told me before. If you're not on schedule, you'll be left out. All right, there's the two sides of this. You have to live here as a person with a severe enough situation that keeps you from living in the outside world. And to know what goes on here day after day, week after week, month after month—then you know the reality.

Despite the challenge of balancing the institutional with the personal, the AL offers services to a population that needs them, and the benefits are huge. For a challenged group of older adults, AL provides a safe environment where their daily care needs are met, most significantly, meals, bathing, and medication. The softer institutional framework of the AL allows these needs to be met efficiently and economically, and flexibility within each setting provides for a degree of adaptation within or modification of its policies to respond to personal preferences and varying needs. However, with these benefits come costs: lack of privacy, limits to independence, spending down one's savings, and less control over one's day. In other words, residents (and, potentially, their relatives) are paying for the privilege of living a soft institutional life. Control is not total; choices, though limited, are offered; independence is compromised but not eliminated; individuality is recognized but impossible to embrace. Unlike Goffman's concept of the total institution, which is all encompassing, the soft institution is sufficiently malleable to incorporate degrees of choice and autonomy. The older adult's care is monitored within some semblance of home.

Quality in an institution, then, involves finding the balance between needs and wants, between what is important and what will be ignored, between what can be manipulated and what is a solid tenet. A soft institution allows this to happen. Mr. Dugan is balancing his daughters' concerns about his health with his friendships with staff and residents. Mr. Granier accepts oversight, because he is able to live in his old neighborhood and has the freedom to drive. Dr. Styles appreciates the flexibility in rules, degree of autonomy, and the willingness of Greenbriar's staff to work with his needs and interests. He has decided not to move into the continuing care retirement community, which was his first choice for relocation, but to make the Greenbriar his permanent home in his retirement.

REFERENCES

Goffman E. (1961). *Asylums*. New York: Doubleday.
McKean, E. (Ed.). (2005). "institution *n.*" [Definition]. *The New Oxford American Dictionary* (2nd ed.). Oxford University Press. *Oxford Reference Online*, Retrieved from http://www.oxfordreference.com/views/ENTRY.html?subview=Main&entry=t183.e39207

3
A Culture of Caring

ORIENTING POINTS

• Residents value emotional and spiritual aspects of care as essential to quality in assisted living.

• Expectations of staff and their roles affect residents' perceptions of quality.

• High, competing demands on staff time present a challenge to fully compassionate care.

• Resident attitudes and behaviors inevitably shape staff performance, thereby influencing quality.

DIRECT CARE STAFF AND THE ESSENCE OF QUALITY

Perceptions of quality in assisted living (AL) depend largely on interactions with direct care workers—those whose job it is to provide for a resident's most physically intimate needs and whose daily presence contributes a significant portion of residents' social interaction. This chapter explores the underlying complexity of quality, as revealed through AL residents' day-to-day encounters with direct care staff. In the stories presented here, residents identify the deeper interpersonal aspects of care that bring comfort to their lives in AL, over and above regulatory or pragmatic requirements. Staff members reveal how the interpersonal aspects of their work bring meaning and purpose to their difficult jobs. While values such as showing respect and maintaining dignity remain central to the philosophy of AL, this chapter addresses aspects of quality beyond the officially stated mission. Personal warmth, sensitivity, and spirituality, especially at the end of life, are widely viewed by residents, family members, and administrators as essential to quality in AL.

At the same time, this chapter also illustrates how multiple and often contradictory demands upon staff make it difficult or impossible to consistently provide care that is truly compassionate. Inadequate staffing levels reduce the capacity of workers to respond quickly to calls for help and engage in meaningful conversation with residents, while low pay and high staff turnover disrupt morale and continuity in care. In some instances, differences in culture or language create misunderstandings that affect staff members' communication with management, residents, and their families. This chapter reveals how some, though not all, direct care workers, despite these challenges, approach their jobs with a sense of meaning and purpose, bring comfort to residents in their care, and serve as exemplars of quality care in AL.

"NO ONE DIES ALONE"

At St. Brigid AL, the Roman Catholic nuns work to ensure that no one dies alone. Staff and residents alike share in the practice of sitting with those approaching death, and they speak of this work as a privilege. Attending to the emotional and spiritual needs of individuals at the end of life generates compassion and comfort that residents, their families, and staff associated with quality care in their interviews. In this story, resident Eileen Wilson describes in detail the experience of sitting with the Sisters while they tended to a priest who was dying:

> And yesterday, I had the privilege—one of the nuns came [into the chapel] and said that Father—the priest that lived here—he was very sick and old—said that he wasn't going to last too long and wanted that nun to come over and sit with him. So that nun, Sister Teresa, said to me, "Come on. Do you want to go with me…and we sit with Father and pray?" So I went. And I went in his room and there was another nun who also went there.
>
> So there were four of us, Ann, Teresa, and the other one whose name I don't know. And there was me, there were four of us in there. And so that was the first time that I had ever been that close to someone who was about ready to die.…
>
> So Sister Ann said to one of the nuns, "Keep a close look on him because he's just got a few minutes left.…" I was so happy to be so close

to this priest who was dying—a good holy man. I didn't know him that much because I hadn't been there that long, but everybody was telling me all the different things he did during his lifetime and kind of the way he helped people and all that. So I was so happy to sit there....

So, finally it came that a nurse walked in and she probably figured that he was already gone.... Well, I was right there holding his hand, can you imagine?

In telling this story, Ms. Wilson emphasized what the Sisters told her—that even though this man was a priest, everyone receives the same sort of care at St. Brigid. Referring to the spiritual care that is offered in the AL she directs, Sr. Mary Catherine explained,

At the end of their life, the Sisters surround them day and night, while they are dying—all through the night, all through the day until—you know we've gotten to where we kind of know and when we see a big change we get all the Sisters together and we see them away together. It's one of the things that the residents look forward to—is knowing the Sisters are going to be there.

In contrast, a disgruntled resident in a different AL lets us know about the noncaring attitude she has observed. *"They'll just let you die in your bed,"* she said.

Residents recognize the value of compassionate care when it occurs, just as they take note when it is absent. For Ms. Wilson, the compassionate end-of-life care offered at St. Brigid contributes to her perception that it is a quality place. As she explained, *"I'm so glad that I looked into this earlier, because I'm already here and I can do for myself. But when that time comes, I'm all ready for them to look after me."* Her needs, wants, and preferences fit well with the profile of what St. Brigid offers, and are in balance with its approach, environment, social context, and services.

ELEMENTS OF COMPASSIONATE CARE

The story that Ms. Wilson shared about end-of-life care at St. Brigid illustrates several elements of compassionate care: human touch and interpersonal warmth, sensitivity in performing body care, and having someone to talk with, as well as a philosophy of care, such as spirituality at the end of life. Although these aspects of care do not necessarily constitute a universal preference, they reflect fundamental elements of quality voiced by a number of residents and their families, as well as staff, in a variety of settings over the course of this study.

It is our work at St. Brigid that led us to first identify the expression of comfort and emotional care as central to quality. Because St. Brigid is much more intentional about its mission to care for and comfort residents in a spiritual and emotional sense, and because the residents there tend to want this sort of care and talked freely about it, there are many examples from this AL in the pages that follow. There are also numerous other examples across settings. Although the staff at the nonreligious settings may not have taken a vow to attend to residents' spiritual and emotional needs, we observed a number of workers doing so nonetheless. In these small personal interactions, beyond the routine tasks of the day, we perceived a deeper meaning of quality.

Truly compassionate care extends beyond the requirements of adequate bathing, nutrition, mobilization, and other care needs for which individuals often move to AL, to the less tangible domain, less attended to by regulators and some owners and managers. Compassionate care addresses the psychological and spiritual needs of the residents. Although the elements of compassionate care described here represent a certain ideal, this chapter also depicts the challenges to providing this type of care, and, together with the information presented in Chapter 8, suggests recommendations for overcoming these barriers.

Human Touch and Interpersonal Warmth

Above all, compassionate care involves human touch and interpersonal warmth, where people connect person to person and feel recognized as individuals. Signs of affection between staff and residents often bring comfort to both. Over the course of this study, we have observed a range of affectionate gestures between residents and staff: a pat on the arm, a hug, or the expression that someone is their "favorite" caregiver or resident. Mr. Braun, a resident of Winter Hills, noted that "associating with the people who work here" makes for a good day. He told us that someone always brings him the newspaper at breakfast, and he regularly speaks with the staff and the "operators," by which he means the directors. He feels a sense of comfort as a result of the warm and personal attention he receives at Winter Hills. These qualities, in the words of Ronni Stinson, whose mother resides at St. Brigid, create a "very loving atmosphere" and signify "genuine concern" for the well-being of the residents.

Residents truly appreciate comfort when they experience it. Staff members, in turn, recognize that this sort of care is mutually beneficial. When asked about the greatest rewards of her job, Pauline, a housekeeper at St. Brigid, replied:

> I'm so rewarded when I see a smile, when I see that I've made them happy, when I leave and do something as simple as find the station on the radio…and they say, "You are wonderful.…you're so special, thank you so much."

Staff member Sule at Wetherby Place approaches his work similarly, "For me, when I come to work in the morning, first thing…I greet them nicely and keep a smile on my face. And it makes most of the residents feel a little bit happier, you know, just talking to them."

Another exchange, the presentation of small, personal gifts between residents and staff, while not permitted in certain settings, symbolizes to some the meaning of these relationships. One resident gave a crocheted stole to a staff member she particularly liked. Tara, who works at Arcadia Springs, spoke about the enjoyment she gets in hearing stories from the residents about what life was like when they were young. "You learn things," she said, "And they learn from us. I mean, this lady right here just moved in. She has the Internet, and she wants us to help her—show her how to use it. And it's just fun that we can help her, and at the same time she helps us with her little stories. So it's nice."

Particular staff members value the personal connections they make with residents and put forth the extra effort to provide comfort. Mrs. Hite, who lives at St. Brigid, shared this story:

> *Like I say, they're all very caring—the Sisters. They go right out to try to help you and comfort you.… And even the helpers. Yesterday, I was all upset about my prescriptions, you know, and I was crying on the lady's shoulder; and then the Sister came last night, and I'm crying on her shoulder.*

This sort of personalized contact and comfort mirrors, from the staff perspective, the benefits of the care described in Ms. Wilson's vignette earlier in this chapter about support and presence at the end of life.

Sensitivity in Performing Body Care

Compassionate and personalized care also involves sensitivity in performing body care. Direct care workers assist with some of the most intimate physical needs of residents. Complaints about "rough handling" and lack of responsiveness to body care needs stand in contrast to other comments heard in this research complimenting the sensitivity of staff. Residents appreciate kindness and humor in these situations. According to Mr. Braskey, who lives in Wetherby Place,

> *I got into a couple accidents [with continence]...unable to control myself. And I thought, "Ugh." They cleaned me up so well, and they laughed and kid with me all the time, and I thought, "Man, how do you accept a messy job like that, and still keep your humor?"...I couldn't do that.*

One son, Mr. Portoni, whose mother is at Boxwood Gardens, observed: "Mother will tell me what bothers her is they're doing something involving her physically without speaking to her beforehand, telling her what's going to come." This same son went on to describe the necessity for gentleness:

> Their answer to everything is, "Oh, at that age the skin is very thin...." Periodically it looks like she's been worked over...and I immediately go to [the Administrator]. I don't believe that they're willfully trying to harm her or anything like that. But it's carelessness—where they grip instead of lift, and you know the distinction between the two. You're going to have a different pressure with the first one.

On the other hand, resident Kathy Moyer, also at Boxwood Gardens, observed that when the aides work with some of the women's hair, the residents really seem to enjoy it. *"It makes them feel better,"* she said. Mrs. Moyer has also noticed staff members helping residents with their clothes and their accessories. Similarly, Anna Salgueiro, who lives at St. Brigid, appreciates compliments from the staff on her appearance, something that is important to her.

Someone to Talk With

For many residents, having someone to talk with is important to feeling contented day-to-day. Opportunities to develop friendships with other residents may be limited due to their neighbors' hearing loss or cognitive decline. In these situations, staff members fulfill the need for human interaction and connection. We have witnessed in our research the development of relationships among residents and staff members who come to know each other on a personal level, simply through regular chats during daily care, transportation to meals, or spare moments. For example, Peter Granier at the Greenbriar enjoyed talking with the Community Outreach Coordinator, who always made time to see him: *"Whenever I felt down in the dumps I would always go. If she was in—you know she goes out on the road a lot—I would go down and sit and talk, and she always listened."* Similarly, Camille Rallings from Wetherby Place has a staff member she can talk with regularly, and she described how this made her feel:

> **Ms. Rallings:** *He is so friendly, and not long ago I was worried about something about my stepson and I said, "Ben, would you sit down a few minutes and talk with me?" and I told him about it. And he explained to me, he said, "Don't worry," he said, "He'll be all right."*
>
> **Researcher:** So you feel like you've got a meaningful relationship.
>
> **Ms. Rallings:** *Oh, yes, yes.*

In contrast, Millie Fischer identified the lack of ample time for staff to sit and talk as a deficiency at Murray Ridge; other residents there were satisfied in this respect, once again showing how expectations and priorities differ among residents.

Staff members themselves recognize how significant it is to take time to talk and get to know residents. In the words of Margaret, a licensed practical nurse who worked at St. Brigid,

> **Margaret:** Just sit there and listen, you know? That means a lot to them, too. Sometimes you just pat them on the shoulder or hug them; that means a lot to them. And you would be surprised what it does.
>
> **Researcher:** So is it a challenge, then, to find ways to do that?
>
> **Margaret:** No, that's not a challenge because, I mean—well we're not supposed to call them sweetie, or honey, or whatever. But, you

know, sometimes you just give them a little pat on the shoulder, do
little things for them, maybe like cut their nails or paint their nails,
listen like I said, listen or talk to them, you know? That helps them.

For residents with more extensive emotional or psychological
needs, professional care may be indicated. However, Medicare will
pay for psychiatric care only in a crisis (Abrams & Young, 2006).
Staff members frequently fulfill the ongoing human need for daily
social interaction, even just in casual conversations. According to
Beth at Winter Hills, "You spend 8 hours a day, 40 hours a week with
these residents and, for some of them, that's all they really do have,
is us."

Philosophy of Care

Compassionate care addresses the emotional and spiritual needs of the
residents, usually reflecting a particular philosophy of care, regardless
of whether the setting is privately owned, part of a chain, or religiously
owned. One staff member, Margaret, at St. Brigid, noted that across the
places where she has worked, she has seen a difference in philosophy
between facilities that are religiously oriented and those that are not.
She stated,

> It doesn't necessarily have to be Catholic. It can be Jewish or
> whatever, it's just that there is a stronger foundation of ownership
> and pride, you know?...Here they hire anybody, any religion or
> whatever, but it's just [here at St. Brigid], we know as employees we
> have to respect the dignity of the elderly the way the Sisters view it.

According to Sister Barbara, a unit supervisor and the activities
director at St. Brigid, the spiritual mission of the organization means,
essentially, "To care for the residents in a special way, trying to bring
God's love to them, you know, and cheer their hearts....Encourage
them along." Similarly, administrators at the nonreligiously based settings sometimes stated their mission in terms of creating a "homelike"
or "family-like" environment, which represents another form of personalized, compassionate care in AL. According to Elizabeth, a direct
care worker in Boxwood Gardens:

Some of them miss their family, even though we are here. And you tell them this is their home; they telling you it's not their home. Because, I think the thing is, some of them, their family does visit them regularly and some of them their family doesn't really come to see them, like they're supposed to. And that kind of frustrates some of them. You know, sometimes they be in a good mood and sometimes not, because they just looking for their family. They asking you, you know, "Where's my son?" or "Where's my this?"— you know, because they don't see them.

Among those we interviewed, it was clear that many staff members recognize the important roles that they play in helping residents deal with emotions like loneliness in AL.

Emotional and spiritual care is especially meaningful at the end of life, as illustrated in the opening story. Similarly, Nancy Wells, whose mother was a resident of Winter Hills, commented on the extra care offered to residents and their families during difficult times:

There was, early on when my mother was there, there was a resident who was dying; she was under Hospice care. The marketing director came with a plate of cheese and crackers and grapes, and whatever she could find to give to the family who was there waiting for the family member to die.

Clearly, such steps are recognized and remembered as especially sensitive, creating a sense of quality. Ms. Wells continued to describe how the nursing staff at Winter Hills attended to the emotional needs of another couple, as one partner was dying:

And in Mr. Braun's case, and I can say it because he talked about it so openly the last few days of Mrs. Braun's life, they moved Mrs. Braun [who had previously lived apart in the dementia care unit in Winter Hills] into his room...so that they could be together. And so she died in that room. I think that was enormously helpful to Mr. Braun, and I think it was enormously comforting to Mrs. Braun, even though she was cognitively impaired.

The Griers, a couple who live together at St. Brigid, noted that the nuns, "*whenever you need anything....they're always there.*" Mrs. Grier stated, *"They're wonderful. It's a miracle to me,"* and Mr. Grier finished her sentence: *"You cannot say enough about this."* The Griers attribute this goodness to the nuns:

> **Mr. Grier:** No, it's they are—they're just wonderful. You couldn't believe—it's really hard for anybody that's been in a nursing home to believe that we could be treated as well as we are.
>
> **Mrs. Grier:** And they make sure that all the help that they hire are the same. If they ever find any that are hollering or anything, they'll give them one good talk and if they do it twice, they're fired.
>
> **Mr. Grier:** They're gone.

Another resident at St. Brigid, Mr. Leland, described the religious setting this way:

> And they mean well, that's another thing—it's not like this place is in it for the money. That's another reason—I agreed [to move here]. My brother got this place, because nuns and everything, being Catholic and, you know, they're not in it to make money. They're in it to help people, and that's what they try to do.

Clearly, this resident has confidence in his AL setting due to its philosophy, based in its spiritual mission, and equates this mission with quality. In other settings and to different residents, the philosophy of care is not as evident as it is in these examples, and challenges exist in the delivery of care that is truly compassionate.

STAFF ROLES AND COMPASSIONATE CARE

Members of AL staff face a number of demands that challenge their abilities to provide the compassionate care described earlier. In part, these challenges revolve around two fundamental and competing orientations in AL: the medical model and the social model. AL encompasses elements of both models, and this dual purpose makes the jobs of the staff more complex. Whether these settings are viewed as primarily medical or social by residents, their families, staff, and administrators can affect perceptions of quality.

Complexity of Staff Roles: Is AL a Medical or Social Setting?

As discussed in Chapter 1, there is a lack of consensus as to how much AL is intended to serve advanced medical needs, which are part of the medical model, compared to social needs. Direct care staff in AL are charged with carrying out a range of daily duties in meeting both personal care and health-related needs of the individuals residing there. Typically, these services include assistance with activities of daily living (e.g., mobility), personal care (e.g., bathing and grooming), and medication administration. Even if residents do not need all of these services when they arrive at AL, they may come to need them as they age in place. A staff member, Gae Wynn at Boxwood Gardens, whose aunt also lives in the setting, explained, "It gets to a point where a resident stays a length of time in this kind of complex [and] they start to get elderly." As they begin to need more help physically and mentally, she continued, they or their families realize that "assisted living is not a medical complex." This realization can affect perceptions of quality, because most do not wish to relocate, particularly to nursing homes.

At the same time that these health needs must be routinely met, social activities constitute an important part of what AL offers, and many residents and their families evaluate quality in terms of the types of activities and social opportunities available. Some residents and their families express disappointment when the social aspects of daily life are neglected. Staff members work to meet social needs through scheduled activities and outings, often for residents who vary greatly in cognitive and physical functioning. As a result of the complexity of their roles in AL, members of AL staff handle multiple, competing demands over the course of an average workday, attempting to fit compassionate care around a demanding routine of care for multiple residents, activities, and meals.

In this regard, expectations differ about what the primary roles of staff should be, medical or social. As described in Chapters 1 and 4, Ms. Carson, when asked what she thought Boxwood Gardens would be like before she moved in, discussed her expectation that the direct care staff would have a higher level of knowledge about basic health. Clearly, this resident is using a medical model to evaluate quality in the setting. Similarly, a researcher on the project recorded the following fieldnotes after speaking with Mr. Portoni, the son of a resident in Boxwood Gardens, who, earlier in the chapter, expressed his concerns about the rough treatment his mother sometimes received:

> Mr. Portoni commented that his mother was much more agile and walked with a walker when she came to the facility. Now he is trying to get the staff to use the walker more with her and get her to practice walking. He does not like the fact that the staff has allowed her mobility to decline, and implied that it is easier and faster for the staff to place his mother in the wheelchair. He is hesitant to assist her, because he's afraid of a fall. He feels the resident care aides should be trained in this. . . . He has asked one of the resident care aides to walk her down to breakfast, as it is served right on her floor. He remarked that he is afraid that some of the staff may be untrained, so he doesn't know how much to push on this issue.

Mr. Portoni expected the staff to take responsibility for his mother's health by encouraging her to walk. With disappointment, he observed that "They get her up in the morning, put her in that chair, and they'll leave her there." He, too, would be happier with an approach that more closely follows the medical model.

In contrast to the views of residents and family who emphasize the medical model, others perceive quality as based in the social aspects of care, such as the courtesy and friendliness exhibited by direct care staff and the types of activities provided. When they move in, some residents look forward to social opportunities in AL, and feel more or less satisfied depending on how well the setting fulfills these expectations. For some, the cheerfulness and responsiveness of the staff become a metric of quality. Ms. Wilson shared this observation of the staff at St. Brigid, "All they have to do is see somebody that needs some help and there's somebody there." She was also impressed by the fact that the nuns eat dinner every night with the residents in the same dining room. They say grace and sit together. Ms. Wilson views the nuns' participation in evening meals as evidence of their commitment to the residents, and this clearly contributes to her sense of quality.

Similarly, Victoria Jones, the administrator of Winter Hills, noted that a good day in AL for residents depends on "interaction on a daily basis with staff," when "staff take the time to say good morning," and when residents "feel like someone cares." Victoria discussed the importance of "having someone to touch your hand, ask you if you want coffee, and make small talk with you." Joyce Henderson, the administrator of Arcadia Springs, also described the significance of close relationships between staff and residents:

> *Joyce:* In the days of my going to school, we were taught, you know, you don't form relationships with your residents. You don't form relationships with people, you just don't do that. That's considered unprofessional. But in this type of setting, one of the things that helps and that makes this work is because the residents do form relationships with the staff and the staff form relationships with them.
>
> *Researcher:* And what are those relationships like?
>
> *Joyce:* They're usually very caring folks. Some of them [staff], you know, you'll hear them call certain residents granny, or [call a] certain resident Uncle this, or Uncle that, you know, whereas that just wouldn't be allowed in a lot of other places. You have to be maintained as Mr. or Mrs. But a lot of our residents, in addition to having just their physical needs cared for, really need to know that somebody is emotionally connected to them.

For many direct care workers, however, it remains a daily challenge to address the physical and health-related needs of residents while also fulfilling their social and emotional needs. One staff member, Tara, described the dual nature of her work at Arcadia Springs this way:

> *Tara:* I'm a CNA [Certified Nurse Assistant] and a med tech, so I'm either on the floor or I'm on the [medications] cart. I either do direct care, helping with the patients, helping them get dressed, helping them bathe, help administer medications, also assist with activities sometimes; and I'm there to be their friend, to be their companion and talk to them—help paint nails, help [do] their hair, any little extra touch that makes them feel good.
>
> *Researcher:* So when do you have time to do those extra things?
>
> *Tara:* We have down time. So when I have my down time and I'm not doing anything else with them, there are a few residents that you find yourself, I guess you could call it closer to, and.... you go into their room and talk to them, and they appreciate it.

The extra time that staffers find to attend to residents equates to what many residents and families perceive as quality, going above and beyond the immediate duties of the job. The inherent duality of this job is managed easily by some staff members, but represents a greater challenge to others, particularly when other challenges derive from the work environment.

Organizational Challenges to Providing Quality Care

The reality of work every day in AL presents challenges to providing care that is perceived as truly compassionate. Specific challenges relate to staffing levels, scheduling, training needs, cultural and language differences, and resident diversity with respect to different physical and cognitive levels and individual preferences.

Staffing Levels

Direct care staff frequently experience the stress of working in a place with minimal or inadequate staffing levels, which may result from high turnover, people not showing up to work, or a corporate decision to reduce staff to improve profits. One staff member, Josephine from Greenbriar, described staffing levels at her AL in this way:

> The biggest challenge is shorting [sic] of staff. You have to work by yourself, give medication and at the same time, make sure the residents are not falling. You have to do more than your tasks, more than your job description. That's the biggest challenge.

In this environment, there may be little time to stop for a reassuring hug or to listen to a resident's story. Aides say they will be "right back" but forget and leave the resident waiting indefinitely. As discussed in Chapter 2, Ms. Carson, a resident of Boxwood Gardens stated, "*I didn't expect all this running in and out. Of saying, I'll be back—but never coming back.*"

Another resident, Mrs. Pollock in Boxwood Gardens, stated that although the staff have been "*overly nice*" with her, she doubts that everyone receives the "*same treatment*," perhaps because they do not speak out as she does. She said:

What I would change is I would like to see them take care of the people that are here for assistance, because they really do suffer. I know two of them, sometimes they forget to bring [one of them] down [for meals]. She doesn't have the use of her legs—but she has her mind and everything.

This quotation evokes a particularly poignant image of a resident suffering because staff had forgotten her, presumably because they had so many other residents for whom they were responsible, and Ms. Kolovos described how her neighbor in Arcadia Springs became so frustrated one night when she couldn't get any help that she called 911.

As acuity levels (the levels of severity of illnesses) have risen in recent years, workers in AL face even higher demands to meet the needs of residents entering these settings. Increasingly, residents arrive in AL with a higher level of health and cognitive impairments (Samus et al., 2009). Both low pay and high staff turnover exacerbate the problem of sustaining a cadre of highly motivated staff to meet the requirements of operating effectively. During the time we spent in these settings, we observed considerable turnover, as well as the termination of problematic staff (see also Chapter 7).

Turnover is well over 50% per year in recent studies of AL staffing and approaches 90% per year in some settings (Castle, 2006); we saw dramatic differences in turnover levels across the settings in our study. One staff member, remarking on a colleague at Arcadia Springs who had been there for 13 years and another colleague who had been there for 5 years, told us: "That's a long time to stay in a place like this, when you're really not moving up," a reflection of the limited career ladder for direct care workers in AL. Whereas some turnover occurs as staff members "move up" by returning to school to train for jobs as licensed practical nurses or registered nurses, others leave staff positions in AL for similar-level jobs in retail or in restaurants.

Although staffing levels remain important, quality involves a dimension beyond the numbers conveyed in a staffing ratio. Quality reflects an attitude, an orientation, an ethic, and is made more difficult to achieve in a short-staffed environment. To illustrate this point, a vocal family member, Mr. Portoni, described a situation in which his mother's roommate was not eating. He witnessed the staff member's behavior, and then intervened himself:

The aide said, "Amelia, Ms. Amelia, come on you haven't had anything. You've got to have something. Can I get you some food?"

"No." It was, no—the answer was no. I happen to know that Amelia doesn't like ice in her beverage. She will not drink it—it will agitate her, so why should you agitate her? I said, "Amelia, will you do me a favor? How about us fixing the apple juice the way you like it, without that silly ice?" [Amelia said,] "Oh, yes, that sounds good." You could connect with the folks—it's not, "Oh it's going to work, regardless, whether you like or…" but you've got to expect that. I got her to the dining room table in the main room, sat down, we poured the juice for her, unwrapped the half of the sandwich, handed it to her, and—[Mr. Portoni, directed to his mother] Right, Amelia ate the last of it. She was hungry. You're right, she was.

Had the staff been more familiar with this resident's individual preferences, and had they had enough time to really understand her needs, they would have been able to more effectively encourage her to eat. In the words of Regina, a direct care worker in Boxwood Gardens, "It's never enough time in a day to give people what I feel like everybody deserves here. It's never enough hours in a day." Limited staffing in long-term care reduces the care that people receive to just a bed and body, to basic minimums, leaving relatively little time for psychosocial care (Henderson, 1995).

Scheduling

Another challenge to quality has to do with the way workers are scheduled, or assigned duties. In the settings we observed, the aides usually rotated across floors or units, and they did not always care for the same residents. From the perspective of the administration, this method of scheduling increases staff familiarity with a variety of residents and provides a wider range of experience for the staff. From the perspective of residents, however, interacting with so many different caregivers can lead to frustration. For example, Ms. Carson, a resident of Boxwood Gardens, complained about having a different care aide every day: "…ever since I've been here, they keep rotating people around. I never know who's going to be coming into my room, or when." When this occurs, the resident feels that no one on staff knows her personally. For the staff member, with so many different residents to care for every day or each week, it is not easy to remember names or special preferences that might personalize both care and conversation. A person is reduced to "just a body," with needs driving requirements for care.

Mr. Portoni has been active in encouraging the administrator to assign the same couple of staff members to his mother:

> And if they [the staff] don't have to continually deal with eight different faces because of the scheduling, and they'd only have to deal with four [in the dementia care unit], it's going to be better for the provider here as well as the receiver that is here. I mean it speaks to respect. They have made inroads on that. Right now—I just checked today—we've got one person who is now assigned to this segment of the facility during the daytime, and at least one for the evening. The second one may be a different face a lot, but there's at least that degree of stabilization, which has got to be a comfort level for any human being. And I know it works much better for Mom, too. They get to know each other, number one. You know, in a large facility you know, there is the book way of doing everything and then there's the actual delivery. And you have to have the skill to augment the book procedure.

From the perspective of some direct care staff, it is difficult to develop personal relationships, to truly understand the needs and preferences of the residents, unless they take care of the same residents every day; and yet, staff rotation remains common.

Training

A further challenge to quality exists in the inadequacy of some training programs and in-service classes, according to some residents' views, and in the failure of supervisors to reinforce what is learned in training on a day-to-day basis. Ms. Carson observed that "*The resident aides should know what's going on. They deal with us constantly.*" However, they have "*no education*" and they "*need training.*" Referring to the lack of regular contact with registered nurses and medical doctors affiliated with the setting, Ms. Carson indicated, "*People with appropriate knowledge aren't acquainted with us.*" This insufficient direct contact with practitioners clearly reflects Ms. Carson's view that AL is primarily a medical care setting.

Training is especially important to staff caring for residents with dementia, and for addressing emotional needs (Tilly & Fok, 2007). Sometimes the staff are faced with frustrating incidents—a resident's lack of compliance, for example. Renee Waller at Arcadia Springs shared the insight she gained through a staff training program:

> Sometimes we have a resident that don't want to take a shower. We just keep being persistent, and they just—you make them mad, so you just leave them alone, and let them calm down and try to come back.

Michelle, an admissions coordinator at Boxwood Gardens, noted that the in-service training programs offered in her setting really do help the staff to deal with difficult situations. The training, she said, offers practical strategies for staff to implement, as well as ideas for addressing residents' emotional needs.

> Here are some ways to calm residents.... To dim the lights. To turn the heat up twenty minutes before you ask someone to take their shower, so that they're not cold. To drape a robe over their shoulders, so that they don't feel like they're standing totally naked in front of a stranger. I think that that training allows us to provide the quality care... to help people spiritually and emotionally as well as meeting their physical needs.

Another issue concerns how the best practices taught in training classes actually become part of the day-to-day routines in the setting, reinforced by management. We have witnessed staff who can speak convincingly about what constitutes quality care, based on what they learned in a training class, but they do not truly implement it when faced with a difficult situation, such as toileting a resident at an inconvenient time. Observations in these settings suggest that staff may be trained to "smile at family" when they visit, but may not necessarily treat residents with the same courtesy. Beyond the buzzwords presented in training, supervisors and managers must ensure that the practices learned in classes, many of which may take additional time to implement, are actually performed by staff day-to-day to maximize quality. For example, Samuel Meadows, the Executive Director of Wetherby Place, in describing what he believes to be the culture of excellent care in his setting, believes that quality can be achieved through both collaboration and education:

> *Researcher:* Where do you think that comes from? What creates that culture of excellent care that you have here?
>
> *Samuel:* Devotion to the residents. The staff really feels like, you know, the residents are family members. And that's kind of cultural thing to a point, but they really care for the residents. I think providing the staff with as much education as you can also helps, and holding them to standards when they do something wrong. Not always writing them up or getting them in trouble, but sometimes it's that educating, it's that nurturing piece of come here, let's go over this together. Or, "Hey, Mr. so-and-so has this. I know none of you have seen this before so come on let's go take a look at it together, and we'll work through it together." Trying just to foster teamwork and education.

Language and Cultural Differences

Differences in language and culture among the staff and residents and their families also create challenges to quality. In the settings we observed, immigrants were sometimes hired to meet the growing demand for direct care workers. In these situations, culture manifested itself not only through differences in language but also through differences in behavior, attitudes, and education among immigrants and American-born staff, as well as differences in the care expectations across groups of residents. One staff member, Gae Wynn, a concierge whose relative lives in Boxwood Gardens, commented that the language and cultural differences can be difficult for the residents:

> It is difficult for a lot of the residents to understand the employees, but the majority of the employees are very kind to them. I know for my [relative] I will keep going back to her; she and a lot of the residents, when they get to a certain point, are hard of hearing and you do need to talk very loud, but very clearly and distinct. Often times the employees don't, and that's difficult.

This staff member went on to explain that the accents are especially difficult to understand, especially for those with hearing impairments.

The ability of the direct care workers to communicate effectively is one parameter this staff member, and a notable number of residents, would use in evaluating quality in AL.

On the other hand, a number of residents spoke about the benefits of associating with staff from other cultures. As will be discussed further in Chapter 7, Mr. Braskey, a resident of Wetherby Place, realized that he felt he had become more tolerant through exposure to so many staff members from different countries:

> *Oh, they ask me what I want. Kid with me, talk with me about any subject—and we laugh. I'm very, very attached to them. They get attached to you—and it's a great relationship. It's something you've never had before.... You find out there's differences in them as in the white people.*

As noted in Chapter 1, Mildred Ashman, a resident from the same setting, stated, "*I really do appreciate what they do. It's not an easy job—it's not a high paying job. You know they're not doing it all for the money. Most of them are from East and West Africa.*"

At times, cultural differences become evident even during routine tasks, such as tuning in a television show for a resident. Mr. Portoni, who we have quoted extensively in several chapters, explained that he has observed that the staff of Boxwood Gardens turn on the programs that *they* like, rather than what the residents prefer. He described this as a matter of culture:

> **Mr. Portoni:** I told you they [the AL] had the histories of what their likes are and what their dislikes for every resident. Socially and otherwise—and that was supposed to be taken into account in coming up with individual plans. I don't know how individual any plans are, because I can recite a litany of stuff that is available through Public Broadcasting that can enrich lives and that doesn't happen here, even though it's on the paper. [It] happens if I'm here. As an example, Mother loves mysteries. She likes Agatha Christie, right? Ms. Marple, and Poirot, and Sherlock Homes and Inspector Morse.
>
> **Researcher:** So they don't put that on for her here, if she's up here?
>
> **Mr. Portoni:** They'll tell you—some of the aides, it's [cultural differences.] Some of the aides put on stuff that they like.

Cultural differences also revolve around core values regarding family and multigenerational caregiving. Many staff members have cared for their own relatives, out of love as well as out of a sense of duty. In the words of Josephine, a caregiver at the Greenbriar:

> I used to love my Grandma so much. So when she died, I was so depressed and I just said, "OK since my Grandma is dead, why can't I just continue taking care of old people?" It reminds me a lot of my Grandma, so that really, really helps me—and looking at them, taking care of them makes me think I'm still taking care of my Grandma.

Staff members who have cared for their own parents or grandparents at home bring additional experience and insight to their work, at the same time recognizing that not everyone can provide for their family members themselves.

Differences in Physical and Cognitive Levels

Quality in AL also has to do with addressing individual needs at different physical and cognitive levels. Dealing with resident diversity adds complexity to staff roles and makes it more difficult for them to provide compassionate care and meaningful activities. Family member and staff concierge Gae Wynn at Boxwood Gardens recommended that the AL's activities include a fairly rigorous exercise program for an hour each day, as well as activities "to keep your mind stimulated." For many residents we interviewed, providing adequate activities meant offering "more than bingo," a staple at many of the ALs in this study. Although bingo was beloved by many, as discussed in other chapters, residents often sought more varied, and more meaningful options to fill their days and to provide meaningful social activity with others. A number of residents articulated an interest in greater opportunities for excursions away from the AL for shopping, a meal out, or to run errands.

Other residents discussed the importance of finding a way within AL to pursue the interests they had enjoyed earlier in life, and to help others. Opportunities of this kind, although not sought by everyone, made it possible for some residents we interviewed to maintain a sense of self-identify and purpose. For example, Martha St. John in Boxwood Gardens was engaged in a number of meaningful activities in her residence. Retired from her government career, she took up painting and had produced a growing body of religiously focused artwork for a one-woman show at the gallery of a local church. She initiated having a public bus stop at the AL, because she needed transportation to the "charity boutique" where she volunteered and purchased her own "nearly new" clothing, and she led the daily exercises with an audiotaped routine, watered the flowers, fed and cared for the birds, and sent out dozens of greeting cards. She told us:

> I do the gardening, I do the flowers—I am what I would call, "officer in charge of morale." I mean there's always somebody in charge of morale. Like for a birthday—I pick a little bouquet and give them a hand written note—but giving that little personal touch to them—or if I see something that needs to be done, then I'll do it.

Enabling residents to help their peers enhances the sense of caring in a setting as well as the sense of self-esteem and self-sufficiency of those residents who contribute. While the activities preferred or pursued depend on the individual residents' physical and cognitive functioning, and their prior interests and experiences, effective opportunities to interact with and help others were very important to a number of residents' perceptions of quality.

EXEMPLARS OF COMPASSIONATE CARE

Despite the challenges discussed previously, a number of the AL staff members we interviewed approached their jobs with a sense of meaning and purpose. They contributed to quality by providing compassionate care that produced comfort, both physically and emotionally, for the residents of AL. One of the most important traits of care providers, according to Gae Wynn, both a member of staff and a relative, is to act with patience. Based on her experience, she shared the following observations:

> You have to know how to multitask, and you have to have patience. Because they [residents] will come to you, let's say for instance within an hour, five times with the same question. And if you give them the same answer, it's not going to work. They're going to continue and continue until they forget it. They want their way.

They expect to have—if they ask you for something, they want it right away, and they will get impatient. You have to be kind and patient with them. You cannot lose your patience, or you can't be in this job—especially the job I'm in right now.

This staff member acknowledges that the work she does is "draining," but that the residents, in the end, seem to appreciate her enthusiasm and courtesy.

Staff Orientation Toward Their Work

The orientation people bring to their work in AL reflects both personal attitudes and experiences; these attitudes have a bearing on interactions with residents and their families, as well as with colleagues and managers. Staff orientations also relate to worker motivation and job expectations. Do individuals work for "just a paycheck," or from a personal desire to help others? Work in AL is difficult, demanding, and messy; some staff members treat residents with emotional distance, limiting their personal involvement, sometimes with the blessing of management. Others display the attitude that personal attention or performing extra services are "not my job." Such attitudes, however, can be found among workers across many careers, limiting their work efforts to only those tasks and deadlines specified by managers. Some use cell phones excessively for personal matters during work tasks or watch television on the job—some seek refuge in residents' rooms to take an "informal break." Some staff members behave carelessly; for example, one accidentally threw a resident's dentures away in the trash. Although all jobs have workers who perform the minimum amount of work with limited care, the implications of this in AL are severe in terms of quality of daily life for residents.

One resident of Boxwood Gardens, Kathy Moyer, offered this assessment: *"There is a set group of people who are caring people, wanting to help,"* and another set that are *"strict and too strong."* Several of the staff were reported to have verbally attacked residents. Ms. Moyer said, *"You know, the way that they talk. I can't tell you how powerful that is."* Not only did some staff members *"yell,"* according to her experience, but *"the higher level [management], too,"* and sometimes, she says, they *"take away their caringness."* She called some of the staff members "*nasty*," although she acknowledged that "*other staff members are nice.*" Another resident, Ms. Rosenstein from Wetherby Place, described her frustration with waiting for unresponsive staff.

> **Ms. Rosenstein:** *When you call them [staff] on the phone, you wait 20 minutes. Suppose I'm having a heart attack, or suppose I fall. I need you. They don't care. To be a nurse means to me, a caring and loving person. They seem to have forgotten that. They're not nurses, they're aides.*
>
> **Researcher:** What would you tell them if you were in charge?
>
> **Ms. Rosenstein:** *I would tell them to stop their giggling, and answer the phone. [When] you call them 2:00 o'clock in the morning—my diaper gets very wet, and I want it changed. So many times I call them....*

Although there may be many reasons for this lack of responsiveness, including low staffing and poor training, the manner in which the staff member responds—for example, with an apology or a sense of concern—can make a major difference in how the resident perceives the incident.

In addition to the physical and emotional demands of this work, the pay in AL is low. For many staff members to persist in this type of work, they must have a sense of purpose or calling. Individuals are motivated to work in AL because of the satisfaction they take in interacting with older people and in helping others. Gail, a caregiver and a supervisor at an AL that participated in an earlier research study, put it this way:

> And that's what I tell a lot of the girls. Care for people has to be a gift from God. You just can't just go into it and say, "OK I'm going to be a nurse." It has to be something that comes from the inside of you, where you have to be a warm-hearted, caring person. Because if you're not, it's not going to work out. You know your resident is going to get neglected. They're not going to be comfortable with you; they're not going to trust you. And there's a point, you want your residents really to trust you and be comfortable with you. So if things do bother them, they can talk to you.

Staff members who have a compassionate orientation toward their work interact with residents in a friendly manner, take initiative to do extra things that are meaningful or special to those in their care, and look for a sense of meaning in their work. To achieve this level of performance, staff must be able to empathize with the needs of those in their care. For example, one staff member we met reflected on the loneliness of the residents in her building, "that maybe nobody comes to visit." Her attitude enabled her to view these individuals as human beings with important needs beyond care of the room and the body.

Some staff members point out that the residents they encounter may not feel well and consider their behavior in that context. A caregiver shared a similar story of how she handles her own reactions to resident complaints or "crankiness." Asked about the biggest challenges that she faces in her job, this staff member, Mariah Brown, replied:

> *Mariah:* I guess some of the attitudes of the residents. Like maybe some days are their off days, so they might be kind of cranky; so that's a challenge for you to be nice and smile and be nice to them.
>
> *Researcher:* Even though they're cranky.
>
> *Mariah:* Yeah. And you don't want everybody looking at you being mean and they think you're a mean person. You still have to be nice regardless of what they do or say.

This staff member displays a caring orientation, remaining calm when dealing with residents who behave unpleasantly. To maintain her composure, she considers her reputation; she does not want to be thought of as a "mean person" by the other staff or residents—or, perhaps, by herself. Another caregiver, Tara, described how she and the other staff members at Arcadia Springs will sometimes talk with one another and offer emotional support during times of stress. When some residents "try her patience," she explained:

> *Tara:* But that's when either you just take a minute, like you know, like "I'll be back," and you take your own private time for a minute, just to get away for a minute, because you don't want to overreact, or say something you don't mean. Just take a minute and take a breather and then come back, or just ignore it because a lot of people here, if they have dementia or Alzheimer's, they don't really realize what they're saying. And it may offend you, but you know what? They don't know what they're saying. Just brush it off, and then you just ignore it. That gets me through a lot of the times, just brushing it off and not worrying about it.
>
> *Researcher:* Do you commiserate then with the other staff here?

> *Tara:* If it gets to the point where I feel like I should talk to somebody, if it gets me that upset, and then our coworkers—we—especially on day shift—we all get along very well. So, if we ever need to talk to one another about maybe a resident, or even a manager or whatever, we get together and we'll talk about it—and we help each other feel better, so that helps.

Yolanda told us that she helps out in tangible ways by doing favors for residents at Arcadia Springs, for example, bringing home their laundry to "personalize it," or running errands. She said that it feels good to provide this sort of kindness and means a lot to the person she is helping. Pauline from St. Brigid described the residents and her work this way:

> Oh, yeah, I do, I love them. I really do. I have a good rapport with them, and, you know, another thing that I learned is that you with the elderly, with the aged, whatever personality they have, you learn to deal with their personality. You deal with their personality, you do. You adjust that day to where they are, because they could be one way yesterday, or even in the next ten minutes. So usually when I say good morning, I can tell from the good morning how far I should take my conversation. Then later on I'll see how they feel.... and if they feel like they may want to, you know, they are all bubbly and they are ready to talk a little, then fine, I do that.

These examples suggest that the interplay between staff and residents, their temperaments, and the orientations they bring to the setting all factor into the quality balance.

Resident's Orientation Toward Staff

The orientation a resident brings to AL, in terms of attitude and outlook, also has a bearing on how quality is enacted. Particular residents stand out because they express concern for their caregivers, complimenting them and acknowledging the difficulty of their jobs. Here, a resident of Boxwood Gardens, Mr. Jones, expresses admiration for a caregiver:

> *Researcher:* Why do you like that first lady?
>
> *Mr. Jones: Because, when she picks out this medicine, she looks at everything. She asks me if you feel good [or] you feel bad. Is there anything*

I can do to help? Now isn't that very, very nice. I think that's the smarts up there [points to head]. That's what I think.

Staff members also feel gratified by such compliments, by acts of kindness, and by thank you notes from residents and family. On the other hand, they sometimes face the challenge of reacting to a resident with a negative orientation. Darlene Hall, the executive director at Murray Ridge, shared this story about a difficult resident:

> And they think it's a hotel, and like you're a maid or something. And even the [staff] tend to get…it's a lot different when you have somebody thanking you all the time, and somebody, you know, expecting it. I mean, yes, it is their job to be here for you; but it's not their job to be griped at. Because this person that I'm talking about, this woman—one of the workers went to the store for her. She wrote up a list, went to the store for her and got everything that was on the list, but everything was wrong. It was the wrong brand, it was the wrong kind, and she threw it in the trash.
> And I said, "Well, don't go to the store for her anymore." It's all I could say. The woman [resident] has five children, so if she asks you go to the store, don't go to the store for her. And if she comes to me, which she will, I'll just tell her that she'll have to get one of her children, because, I mean, they [staff] don't have to go to the store for them. That's—and the girls do go above and beyond. There are a lot of them that go to the store for them. They don't have to go to the store for any of them, you know, but they do.

Residents tend to notice and respect the staff members who do a good job and gravitate toward them. Mr. Portoni, speaking on behalf of his mother in Boxwood Gardens, commented, "You have a few folks that you would love to clone—they're that good. You have others who do the best they can—well intentioned, but lacking in certain areas of effectiveness. Occasionally, you run across those that ought to be in another means of livelihood, and fortunately those get identified, and they move on." A number of residents have told us that when they are treated well, they choose to reciprocate by "being easy" with staff, showing patience for delays, or simply by cooperating and "going with the flow." Residents also offer their compliance and good behavior as a way to give something to staff when they are not permitted to offer presents or tips. This reciprocity exemplifies an important dynamic in

AL. In exchange for the care that they receive, some residents show that they care by trying to make the lives of the staff easier.

In a sense, then, quality in AL relates not only to the orientation of the staff member, but also to the personal characteristics, attitudes, and behaviors of individual residents. When the resident's attitude conveys a sense of appreciation and receptivity to care, it has a bearing on the staff member's attitude and attention in the care that he or she provides to the resident. As discussed in Chapter 1, a resident at Murray Ridge, Eileen Howe, commented, "*It's what we make it, you know what I mean?*" Ms. Howe recognizes that some people "*complain about everything,*" but, she says, "*There's nothing to complain about. . . . I just made it home.*" Ms. Howe has made this setting feel like home by "*bringing family with her.*" She has posted her family photos on the wall, and continues to look for the good in her living situation.

The following anecdote by staff member at St. Brigid further illustrates how resident orientations affect staff attitudes and behavior.

> *Joan:* And there was one resident and her name was Mrs. Lane and she's gone home now and she yelled at me one night. She was funny—[knocking] "Sweetheart, sweetheart," and she'd always call me sweetheart. She called everybody sweetheart, and "my tea is cold." And she really yelled at me, and I just took it to heart and I started to cry. And then I learned to really love that lady more than anybody else here. I mean, and she apparently liked me and she was just a lovely, lovely lady. She really, really was.
>
> *Researcher:* Once you get past the grumpiness?
>
> *Joan:* She always was—but it was like—she didn't mean any harm. So you had to get beyond that, yeah.
>
> *Researcher:* Sometimes those are the people that are so rewarding, once you get to know. . . .
>
> *Joan:* She'd say, "I'll pray for you every night. I'll pray for you going home." I said, "Good," because I hate driving. And she was just a lovely lady and it was like she was a friend of mine, a real good friend of mine.

Although Joan was able to see past this resident's initial behavior, it is difficult for anyone to continue to behave nicely toward someone who persistently speaks or acts in a nasty way. The majority of the staff members we have encountered behaved admirably in this respect. Renee Waller, a medication technician at Arcadia Springs, acknowledged that, fortunately, "[W]e don't have too many residents that are rough and hard to get along with."

TOWARD A CULTURE OF CARING

Although ALs seek to employ skilled, motivated, and compassionate workers, the managers whom we interviewed said that a relatively small number of staff continue in the same setting for years. It remains a challenge to hire, train, and retain direct care workers who find rewards sufficient to compensate for all of the competing demands and the low pay of the jobs. Managers may not be able to greatly increase pay, as that would increase the cost of AL overall, making it less affordable. Clearly, the staff who stay in AL over many years are working for more than money (Ball, Perkins, Hollingsworth, & Kemp, 2010; Ball et al., 2005). Intangible rewards offer the greatest potential to retain workers who bring quality to these settings through compassionate care.

Direct care staff members respond to sincere efforts by management to reward them and make them feel valued. In the experience of Elizabeth Hastings, a staff member at Boxwood Gardens, recognition for her work makes a difference in how satisfied she feels on the job:

> People go to work, it's not only for the money; but you go to work because you want to feel that you are needed. You're there, you're doing your work and, if there's somebody out there that's appreciating you, I mean if your boss can see that you're a good person, why not let you know?

Staff well-being is crucial to providing quality care, and communication is essential. According to Elizabeth, "If you work in a place that people are warm towards you and caring, you know—you want to come to work every day, regardless of the paycheck." St. Brigid offers an annual award to the employee, nominated by the staff, who exemplifies the virtues of the founder of their religious order. The recipient need not be a nun, and receives a party, a special parking space, a plaque, and flowers. "It's quite an honor to be chosen by your staff," according to the director of St. Brigid.

Administrators who speak of the importance of providing compassionate care and reward staff for doing so set the tone for a culture of caring in their AL setting. Administrators shape both the composition of the staff and the priorities of the organization, and there are definite differences in general staff orientations, based on the style and philosophy of the leadership (Eckert, Carder, Morgan, Frankowski, & Roth, 2009). One resident, Eileen Howe, noted that she has never been in a situation in which she needed something and could find no one to respond to her, *"Because they're very particular about who they choose to work here."* Mrs. Howe attributed the responsive care that she received at Murray Ridge not only to the quality of the staff selected to work there but also to efforts to retain them—and, from a staff member's perspective, Pauline at St. Brigid noted, "You have to like what you are doing. [If] you don't have a passion in doing it, you won't give your best, or you won't even enjoy what you're doing."

Administrators look for certain personal qualities in their hiring decisions and then reinforce these values. Darlene, the administrator of Murray Ridge, once worked as a caregiver herself and recognizes what it takes to do an excellent job.

> The staff, they have to have a certain attitude, they have to have a certain patience. To work this every day—to come here every day and work, especially with—downstairs with Alzheimer's—you have to have a certain patience. I mean, there are some people that are not cut out for this place. I mean, I've had employees come in here—they thought they wanted to go into nursing, and wanted to take care of the elderly. Well, they come here and they don't have the patience, so [I] get rid of them. I think that one of the nicest things anybody ever said to me was, I had a family member tell me—and this was when I was in nursing—she said, "[I]f there is a heaven, there is a special place up there for you."

As they go about their daily routines, the care staff enact the vision of the administrators (Mead, Eckert, Zimmerman, & Schumacher, 2005). Martha St. John of Boxwood Gardens offered this advice to management:

> *Really circulate, because—well, I know there are staff meetings and everything—but [when you are circulating] you see things. Make it a point every day to get out of that office....and get to know each of the*

residents. And there's no substitute for that—I know for sure that [the executive director here] confers with all the families. But I think, get out and mingle or come to the dining room or something like that.

When the staff sees the administrators interacting with residents and talking with them, it sets an example for direct care workers to do the same—and, although it seems like common sense, it may not happen as often as intended.

Leaders also have a responsibility to see to it that their staff members view residents as individuals, and that they have opportunities to learn about each resident personally and understand their likes and dislikes, as well as their needs. A number of AL residences have asked residents to submit forms that describe their life histories and preferences. In cases of residents with dementia, family or friends must help to convey this information. With knowledge of their preferences and earlier lives, it becomes easier for staff to view each resident as a person and to provide compassionate care, an essential component of quality. According to Tara, a caregiver in Arcadia Springs,

> I think if the staff knew more, like I think the staff, if we had an exact idea what this person used to be, how they used to be treated, who they were 30 or 40 years ago, I think it would make people look at them and respect them even more. But staff look at them now as how they are now. And it's kind of hard to imagine, like if we could find out what they did in the past, and we knew their life, I'm not saying every detail, but if we knew like the basics of their life, it would be—maybe more people would respect them. Like, "Wow! This person did this and this and this, back in their life. And they deserve credit, no matter what they did, because they survived this world."

COMPASSION AS A CALLING

This research illustrates how particular direct care workers in AL provide truly compassionate care that includes human touch and interpersonal warmth, sensitivity in performing body care, meaningful conversation, and the expression of a philosophy of care such as support and spirituality at the end of life. Despite inadequate staffing, low pay, and changing rules and regulations, many of these workers strive to bring comfort and compassion to those in their care. Such staff members possess an intrinsic motivation, describing their work as a "calling" to help others. They perceive their roles in the setting as meaningful beyond the pay and benefits, and they express a sense of pride in their work. The challenge in AL is to locate workers who possess this internal "calling" to help others, to support them in providing high quality care, and to foster an organizational culture of caring. The interaction between staff and residents, their temperaments, and the orientations they bring to the setting all factor into the quality balance.

REFERENCES

Abrams, R. C., & Young, R. C. (2006). Crisis in access to care: Geriatric psychiatry services unobtainable at any price. *Public Health Reports, 121*(6), 646–649.

Ball, M. M., Perkins, M. M., Hollingsworth, C., & Kemp, C. L. (2010). *Frontline workers in assisted living*. Baltimore, MD: Johns Hopkins University Press.

Ball, M. M., Perkins, M. M., Whittington, F. J., Hollingsworth, C., King, S. V., & Combs, B. L. (2005). *Communities of care: Assisted living for African American elders*. Baltimore, MD: Johns Hopkins University Press.

Castle, N. (2006). Measuring staff turnover in nursing homes. *Gerontologist, 46*(2), 210–219.

Eckert, J. K., Carder, P. C., Morgan, L. A., Frankowski, A. C., & Roth, E. G. (2009). *Inside assisted living: The search for home*. Baltimore, MD: Johns Hopkins University Press.

Henderson, J. N. (1995). The culture of care in a nursing home. In J. N. Henderson & M. D. Vesperi (Eds.), *The culture of long-term care: Nursing home ethnography* (pp. 37–54). Westport, CT: Bergin & Garvey.

Mead, L. C., Eckert, J. K., Zimmerman, S., & Schumacher, J. G. (2005). Sociocultural aspects of transitions from assisted living for residents with dementia. *Gerontologist, 45*(suppl 1), 115–123.

Samus, Q. M., Mayer, L., Onyike, C. U., Brandt, J., Baker, A., McNabney, M.,…Rosenblatt, A. (2009). Correlates of functional dependence among recently admitted assisted living residents with and without dementia. *Journal of the American Medical Directors Association, 10*(5), 323–329.

Tilly, J., & Fok, A. (2007). Quality end of life care for individuals with dementia in assisted living and nursing homes and public policy barriers to delivering this care. The Alzheimer's Association. Retrieved from http://www.alz.org/national/documents/End_interviewpaper_III.pdf

4

Hidden Complexity
Food and Dining in Assisted Living

ORIENTING POINTS

- Dining is a highly valued, socially important "activity" of daily life.
- Food is intertwined in many ways with residents' views of quality.
- Institutional food preparation, cost, and regulations limit the quality of what is on the plate.
- Meal schedules, assigned seating, and narrow menu options limit control and choice over where, when, and what residents eat.

RESIDENT ACTIVIST AND FOODIE

When I came, I was in a state of shock. It was like culture shock.... I certainly expected them to have much more knowledge in basic health and medicine—that was one of the shocks. You couldn't talk to anybody about basic health, because they didn't even understand it. I was shocked by the food, by the nutrition, the unbalanced nutritional meals, that they didn't have a nutritionist. And the person working in the kitchen didn't know what I was talking about—of balanced foods, the fruits and vegetables. I had many shocks.

—Ms. Carson

A retired biologist, Ms. Carson moved into Boxwood Gardens precisely because she needed some assistance and oversight; her health was making it difficult to complete the larger tasks of daily living—keeping house, grocery shopping, preparing meals, and washing laundry. Although not enamored with the move, she accepted her fate. Boxwood Gardens was selected because of its familiar location.

89

Ms. Carson brought her handicapped-modified van and found this community easily accessible and within driving distance of her old neighborhood, church, doctors, friends, favorite vintage coffeehouse, and the nature center where she volunteered.

To say that Ms. Carson is outspoken is an understatement. She is opinionated, with the issues that concern her centering on medical care, healthy eating, and the environment. She took Boxwood Gardens to task for what she called poor medication management and staff attitudes and behavior. To promote a greener environment, she called for recycling, planted native wildflowers on the grounds, and positioned a wren house on a fence outside her window, which she regularly filled with seed.

Healthy food, however, is her top priority. An activist, she sent for information on nutritional requirements for older adults from Tufts University and then reprinted these articles and distributed them to staff and interested residents. She tried talking with the person in charge of the kitchen, whom she found unqualified to head a dining program, characterizing her as more in the food services business than knowledgeable in nutrition. The man in the suite next door, a retired dentist, told her that the material she distributed from Tufts was some of the most interesting information he'd read in quite some time, but the dining services director ignored her.

At the time of our initial interview with her, Ms. Carson had already been advocating healthy eating for 2 years. "*I still don't have that through their heads.*" She had been trying to get the assisted living (AL) to understand the difference between green vegetables and leafy vegetables, and also to offer alternative choices to the main entrée besides cottage cheese and canned peaches. Fresh fruit was rarely offered, but she has learned to ask for bananas to take back to her room. The researcher asked if, over time, Boxwood Gardens had increased their offering of fruit.

> As a matter of fact we're getting less fruits because they don't put them out. They keep some in the kitchen, but you have to go ask for them and you have to know that they are there. But they're supposed to give me bananas, but I have to go ask for them and usually they tell me no. So then I ask another person, because she told me no yesterday. So I asked

somebody else that came out of the kitchen and she said, "We have bananas, but they're not ripe yet." And I said, "That's fine. Give me the unripe bananas and I'll keep them in a bowl, and when they get ripe then I'll have them," because when I've gotten bananas before they had been beyond ripe and they were all squashy—like I used to make banana bread, when the bananas got that way. They really don't know how to take care of bananas. So, I got some up here. She gave me three because I said, "Give them to me anyway." She said, "They're not ripe yet." I said, "Give them to me. I know when they're ripe."

This example of Ms. Carson's experience speaks to issues beyond healthy eating, which make the arena of food and dining so complex. Bananas, as one example, become contested property between resident and staff member; one wants, the other withholds, and this dynamic reflects power and acceptance (see Chapter 6). Few residents are like Ms. Carson, who battles for fresh fruit. More will eat canned peaches or, like Mr. Granier of the Greenbriar, shop on their own for freshness in their food. It bothers Ms. Carson that she spends a lot of extra money buying food that should be provided under her housing contract. Realistically, she doesn't expect Boxwood Gardens to supply her preferred organic soup and juice, but she does expect the food supplied to her and others to have a fairly high level of nutritional quality, rather than the more common pattern of heavily sugared fruits and beverages.

During one of the interviews with the ethnographer, a tray was delivered to Ms. Carson's room. She was upset with a staff member, and dinner was sent to entice her to eat. From fieldnotes:

Ms. Carson got off the couch and went to look at her tray. She got a container of milk and a mushy mixture of what looked like ground beef, tomato sauce, and noodles. She noted that they get a lot of *that* kind of food. She also had slices of yellow squash. She said she would eat the yellow squash, and she hoped it wasn't too buttery. She is trying to get Boxwood Gardens to cook two complementary vegetables per meal, and when I asked about a salad, she said that a salad to them is a slice of lettuce with a spoon of cottage cheese and a canned peach on the top. She also got a dish of peaches with her dinner and said she'll eat some of it, but she's sick of eating canned fruit.

That kind of food refers to a processed diet, in Ms. Carson's view. Another tray observed by the ethnographer in Ms. Carson's suite highlights this concern even more:

> She sent for a lunch tray that came with no milk. For one hour and fifteen minutes, she has had her "buzzer" on, trying to get someone's attention about the milk. Her preference is for skim, but they often don't have it.... The dining room will "likely be closed" by the time the buzzer is answered. She received a sandwich with processed meat and cheese on white bread with canned pineapple.... She ate the cheese and some of the fruit.

Normally Ms. Carson does her own grocery shopping and buys *"cereal, brown bread, fruit, and fresh greens."* She noted, *"As long as I can get up myself...get myself to the grocery store...I am okay,"* but on another day she says, *"I cannot often get out to buy groceries. I cannot often get out to do any of the things I'd like to do. I just don't have the strength and energy anymore that I used to."* Luckily, Ms. Carson has a daughter who is able to do some of the shopping for her, and she does have her van for days during which she feels well enough to go out in search of the foods she believes support her health.

Ms. Carson, after 2 years, notes, *"I've calmed down since I've come,"* but she has not relinquished her identity as an activist.

COMPLEX ISSUES AND MULTIPLE VIEWPOINTS OF FOOD IN AL

Healthy Eating

Although an outlier in an AL, Ms. Carson is right on target with what professionals say about diets of older Americans. In a recent publication, *Older Americans 2010: Key Indicators of Well-Being,* issued by the Federal Interagency Forum on Aging-Related Statistics, an analysis of diet quality showed the significance that nutrition plays in the health of older adults (Federal Interagency Forum on Aging-Related Statistics, 2010). "A healthful diet can reduce cardiometabolic risk factors, such as hypertension, diabetes, and obesity.... Since diet is a modifiable lifestyle factor, dietary improvement can lead to reduced disease risk and improved health in older adults." Although the current average diets are far from debilitating, the researchers determined that "average intakes of saturated fat, sodium, and calories from solid fats, alcoholic beverages, and added sugars were too high and failed to meet the quality standards in both age groups" (ages 65–74 and ages 75 and older). In addition, "to meet federal guidelines, older Americans would need to reduce their intake of foods containing solid fats and added sugars, limit alcoholic beverages, and reduce their sodium (salt) intake. Healthier eating patterns would also include more vegetables, whole grains, oils, and nonfat/low-fat milk products." In other words, Ms. Carson is correct in asking Boxwood Gardens to rethink canned peaches, white bread, and processed cheese.

Across sites, families were especially supportive of nutritious food. A daughter-in-law wondered if residents at Arcadia Springs were hoarding, which would explain why, she commented, "there's no fresh fruit out any more." A daughter found that "vegetables looked overcooked and mushy and you don't get the fresh fruits, seasonal fruits…I think they just have the standard apples, bananas, and oranges." In discussing her father and stepmother, the relative at Boxwood Gardens spoke of a difference between how they ate prior to their move-in and at home, and corroborated the answers in their interview. "They were pretty healthy at home." Here "they don't get like fresh peaches; they get canned peaches, or you know everything is cooked until it's mostly mush." She refers to the food as "pretty standard cafeteria fare."

Families were also concerned about fat and sugar. Gae Wyn, a niece of an AL resident who also works at Boxwood Gardens, noted that:

> …a lot of what they get is full of sugar, condensed food fixed fast and all. See I am very strong on diet and—not that I'm on a diet, but I mean what you eat and I would be very—I'd be more careful of what type of foods they ate and making sure that they all had liquid. That they drank water because often times they do get dehydrated and that onsets another problem, they have to be taken to the hospital and then if they don't drink enough then they get urinary tract infection.

Family members and their resident often disagreed. A daughter of the Griers at St. Brigid commented:

> I don't know the whole story behind why they serve some of the meals they serve, but I don't feel that they are low fat, I don't feel

that [they are appropriate] for heart patients—[there is] a lot of salt in some of the food and I think they could do better with the nutritionist. I see it with my own Dad. He is a diabetic, he needs to be taught.

Yet in two separate interviews, the Griers told our researcher that the food is healthy, which they partly characterized by a "*salad every noontime...soup every night and a light supper.*"

Alternative meals (food offered when the residents dislike the entrée) are also problematic. Mr. Portoni takes issue with the fact that residents are not reminded that they can ask for something else and that all it consists of is "Jell-O or a scoop of cottage cheese and maybe canned peaches or something." He suggests, "Take the vegetable from the main meal they're not eating and just substitute something for their meal," like a fruit plate or a grilled cheese sandwich.

Some residents do concur with Ms. Carson. Ms. McCoy at Arcadia Springs commented that "*in one meal we had corn one day and we had gravy [laugh], which is nuts—I love it myself, but it's not what I would call healthy food.*" Ms. Meisel of Boxwood Gardens finds their food healthy "*if you want to live on cornbread and rolls,*" and Mr. Reichelson, although in the minority, admonishes the Greenbriar for their style of food preparation.

A person of a certain age has to have certain foods to eat. Everything has been fried—the cheapest way—fried fish, fried this, fried chicken, fried—what do you think I need at this time in my life with you frying everything for me? I don't need it.

Then there are residents and family members whose evaluation mirrors those of the Griers, and who find food choices at their respective ALs homes to be healthy. In his interview, Mr. Cohen of Wetherby Place exclaimed, "*[It's] very important. I have diabetes. If the food weren't healthy, I'd be dead by now [laughs].*" A family member notes that in Murray Ridge "they feed them really nice and a nice balanced meal," and some residents assume that the AL settings have "nutritional rules." Definitions of nutrition vary. Ms. Rosenstein "thinks" the meals are healthy despite the fact that she has gained 14 pounds since coming to the AL, though she does attribute this to her daily breakfast of "*egg with bagel and cream cheese, and the cream cheese is so terribly fattening.*" Ms. Carson might not agree with Mr. Benham's notion of nutritious as *"honey roasted pork chop...with some kind of gravy over it,"* though they did have *"baked potato and squash...and a delicious molasses cookie for dessert....Good food."*

A number of residents say that they don't care about eating healthy *"if it tastes really good."* Susannah, Ms. Pollock's daughter at Boxwood Gardens, told our researcher, "I don't care about that any more. What difference does it make at 86 whether it's healthy or not. I mean they get so caught up in that 'healthy' that they don't feed them anything they like."

A son whose dad is a resident at Greenbriar agrees.

> *Ronald:* A lot of people would think the food needs to be healthy, but you know what? The man is 81 years old. We grew up on pork fat, back bacon roasts, over an open fire. They didn't care about cholesterol then, so—if the man wants bacon and eggs, let him have bacon and eggs.
>
> *Researcher:* So at this age, if a resident isn't interested in nutrition...
>
> *Ronald:* Absolutely not, absolutely not. I can remember some of the stuff that he made when we were younger—I can feel my arteries clogging right now. They blame all that high blood pressure, and high cholesterol, on heredity. Blame it on your parents, well, I'm blaming him. Because I got it, too. None of us ever cared about that.

Diverse Preferences

"Do residents like the food in their respective settings?" we as an investigative team wondered. "Was Ms. Carson the only disgruntled resident?" The food at Boxwood Gardens reflects findings at our other research sites and probably the food at most other AL settings. Some residents here like the food; *"The food does very well,"* according to Ms. St. John. Some are *"not enchanted"* with it, whereas others find it *"pretty good."* Ms. Morris calls it *"terrible"* and *"horrible."* Mr. Chase blames the problems with food on collective living, attributing lack of seasoning, and therefore lack of taste, to varied diets prescribed for residents. Ms. Gentile feels the food is *"like any institutional food can be—some you like and some you don't."* Consequently, the residents' responses to evaluating food at their respective settings ran the gamut of *"Cereal is about the best thing in here"* to high praises for menu selections on a daily basis: *"The food is good. It truly is good."*

Individuals do not always move into an AL from their own communities, relocating instead to the towns and suburbs of family members. Therefore, food preparation in the AL will often not reflect their regional cuisine back home or accommodate their religious or dietary preferences. "*Of course Maryland cooking is not like my Kentucky cooking,*" Mr. Benham tells the researcher, and when Ms. Rosenstein is asked if "they (Wetherby Place) cook food the way you used to cook food (at home)," she responds, "*Oh, no. I'm Jewish, this is not a Jewish Home.*" The Moyers, a married couple, remark in their interview about adjusting to life in the AL that "*It's impossible to continue as a vegetarian at Boxwood Gardens....Also, for the Jewish people it's very hard to eat here.*"

We were able to interview chefs at the settings who, not surprisingly, take an active interest in their work. Wendy at Arcadia Springs compares food preparation in a hotel with AL:

> See, in the hotel, you're doing hors d'oeuvres, you know all the fancy stuff, fancy meats, different stuff. But here it's just—how can I put it, it's more personable [geared to the residents living here], you know. It's just home. I mean I cook for them like I cook at home, just without a lot of salt, you know that's it. That's the only difference. Not a lot of seasoning on it, but it's just like at home.

However, despite what Wendy says, we did hear on more than one occasion a response similar to that of a resident's daughter from the same AL where Wendy works: "*No place you live has food like home.*" For some of the residents who were eating poorly before they moved into the AL, this can be construed as a positive response.

Several chefs, like Marie at the Greenbriar, spend time talking with residents and also actively solicit recipes from them to make in their new home. Chefs are also concerned with food preferences and healthy eating. The role the dietary staffs have taken on is to serve wholesome food, gauge residents' preferences, and provide oversight within the larger scope of the rules embedded in the AL.

Corporate's Role

Mr. Jones, who gives Boxwood Gardens high praise generally, attributes some of its lack of culinary success to the business model of AL.

Initially in the interview, when thinking abstractly about food served at a special event, his evaluation was positive: "...*and the food isn't— now this is not a hotel—but the food here is pretty good, and for what you're paying, it's pretty good.*" Giving this more thought, later on in the interview, he commented:

> *It's just fair—it's just fair. Now I have a cousin, his mother and father were in assisted living and he was saying the same thing. The food isn't as good as we thought it would be. But I guess that's the way—after all they're in business to make money. Well, now—so their whole idea is they are the largest corporation to own this, and their idea is to make money. In other words—that's what they're here for—to make money. And I just have to get used to [the fact that] this is the way I'm going to live.*

When the researcher asked what change Mr. Jones would initiate to make life better for residents who live at Boxwood Gardens, he answered, "*I think, the food.*"

Ms. Carson, in her activist mode, also spoke of the influence of the corporate model on food. She met with the "corporate nutritionist," a representative from the company with which Boxwood Gardens contracts for food services. Ms. Carson tells us about that experience.

> *All she did was sit there. And she said, "Well, I've learned a lot, I guess it's time to go." The problem is that she's working for a corporation. That's the whole problem with this place too—it's a corporation. They're out for money; they're not out for help and care. This food—or [food contractor] or whoever they're called is the same as like if you would get when you drive up to an airplane, they put the food on. They put the food out. I don't—I am used to working with academic people. I'm not used to working with business people. I don't really care that much about business as long as people make enough money to live what is an average or a little above average in America or a little below average and have some incentive to make a little more money. I don't agree with capitalism to the point that it's being used by our elderly population. These places are springing up all over the place and how many of them know anything about the body, about health, about symptoms, about personalities, about our emotions? Almost none of them.*

AL settings that are part of corporations are subjected to control by management who are off-site. Menus are distributed to the settings on a fairly regular basis, as recognized and noted by residents. Ms. Brubaker acknowledges that Greenbriar has *"very good cooks,"* but

> *They need a new menu. As a matter of fact, it's like you can almost tell what you're going to get—every other day or so, because it's just the same thing over and over.... It's healthy and that's important...I would like to see who makes the menus up and give them a little piece of my mind because you get tired of the same things week after week, after week, after week. I think the menu should be changed.*

Actually, at the Greenbriar, the dietary staff has some control over the menu. Marie and the director keep track of what the residents consume and reject, and this reflection helps to alter the menus that the corporate office sends out. They get menus in cycles of 4 months, and Greenbriar records what is eaten and also talks to residents, both in the dining room and at Food Council meetings. Corporate does allow changes, as Marie told us.

> When the menus come we see it, then we take something off, put something else. What they don't like...—we take that out,\ ...because we know when you serve the residents, what they eat. If they don't like it, we know it.

The changes may not be enough for Mrs. Brubaker and the other residents at the Greenbriar.

Another issue related to corporate management and food concerns options for residents with dietary considerations—especially diabetes—and diabetic alternatives are a hot button issue for residents. Diabetic residents not only complain about the lack of dessert choices but also note the frequent use of highly sugared sauces, for example, barbecue sauce for ribs. A family member confided that "I'm sure that a lot of people are diabetic and they are giving ice cream to everybody. And they are getting white bread. They are getting stuff that they shouldn't have." In general, and when they are available, three sugar-free desserts tend to be offered to diabetic residents: ice cream, pudding, and Jell-O. Tara, a staff member at Arcadia Springs, has evaluated the situation.

> I think the diabetics get gypped. Residents have these nice big cakes and desserts and the diabetics get fruit. They don't always

want that. I think it would be nice to have the diabetics have a special kind of a special dessert.

We learned from Marie how important dessert is to the residents: "When they come into the dining room, at the beginning of the meal, they ask about dessert first!"

In their respective ways, Mr. Jones, Ms. Carson, Mrs. Brubaker, and Marie acknowledge the bureaucratic nature of AL and the role of the corporation that sustains it. AL is collective living and by necessity and efficiency runs according to internal rules and regulations that provide acceptable care. Boxwood Gardens and the other sites we researched are not boutique residences. They are settings that provide assistance to a diverse group of people with assorted needs who move in with varied incomes and preferences. In addition, these settings are affected by the same economic booms and downturns as other businesses, and a low enrollment (fewer people living at the AL paying the monthly fees) may mean tighter budgets for all aspects of daily life, including the menu. This impacts dietary services and is reflected in what menus are prepared. Consequently, we have observed that the quality of food is affected. For Boxwood Gardens, the Greenbriar, and our other sites, fewer residents and less money means limited options and more canned peaches.

Eating Beyond the Dining Room

In our research, we both saw and heard about a variety of food options aside from the scheduled meals and their alternatives in the dining room. We spotted room refrigerators, microwaves, and shelves stocked with optional food choices, and heard discussions about going out for meals with family and friends, as well as with other residents on field-trips; we even had a research team member retrieve a pizza delivered to Boxwood Gardens during an interview with Ms. Meisel, who ate part of it while talking with her.

While the dining room demonstrates one dimension of food service in AL, there are alternatives, some of which are very important to particular residents or their family members in shaping views of quality. Ms. Meisel is one example as she orders out *"maybe once a week."* After all, *"There's occasions when you want to have Chinese food, when you want to have something different."* However, delivery can become problematic for some ALs because it puts more work on the staff. The researcher who retrieved the pizza for Ms. Meisel wrote this in her fieldnotes:

> I noticed that she [Ms. Meisel] kept looking out of her window. I thought perhaps she was watching the construction workers, but she was, in fact, keeping an eye out for her pizza delivery. When she saw the car drive up, she asked me to get down from a cabinet shelf a container out of which she took a $20 bill. She then asked me to go to the main desk, pick up her pizza, and pay the driver. When I got there, the man was trying to explain to Gae, the concierge, that he was there to deliver a pizza to Ms. Meisel. Gae [concierge] seemed exasperated. I came out with the $20 bill, paid for the pizza, and gave a dollar tip as directed by Ms. Meisel. Gae was not at all pleased with the way this was going. She said that everybody is being used by Ms. Meisel, and Gae implied that there has been quite a bit of trouble and annoyance with this resident.

Residents who enjoy going out of the AL for meals will do so primarily with family or friends; sometimes by themselves, as in the cases of Ms. Carson and Dr. Styles, who drive vans; or with other residents, as is the case with Mr. Granier and Mr. Dugan. The activities director will schedule restaurant field trips for residents who have no such connection and for those who enjoy going out with their acquaintances in the building. But these outings can be very expensive for those on a strict budget, and cumbersome for an activities staffer who needs to coordinate how many residents the AL can take with what specific assistive devices. It was only recently, in fact, that the Greenbriar purchased a bus large enough to transport residents confined to wheelchairs or scooters; earlier, they were left out of field trips. Increased dementia in some ALs may also be a reason why some of them have curtailed trips to public places. In an interview, Ms. St. John, a resident at Boxwood Gardens, told us,

> *Speaking of eating out, my first years here we used to have once a month...a dinner on the town. We would go out to different restaurants...and I found they [some residents] were utterly lost. They couldn't order. They didn't know what to select. And we always said, "These look good." They'd bring a dessert cart around...[one resident] said "I want one of everything." When I realized that was her way of*

covering up, I'd say, "Oh, you like the chocolate pudding. Here you go, chocolate pudding." See, all those little things that we take for granted in a restaurant—lots of them couldn't order. . . . I notice they [Boxwood Gardens] don't go—they seldom go out to eat anymore.

Taking residents on field trips to complicated places is another part of AL life that requires additional staff. Some residences put more effort into the success of this activity than others.

Residents' options related to food are situated mostly within each AL. The dietary staff plan special meals that often coordinate with residents' wishes. Candlelight dinners, Mardi Gras before Lent, barbecues for Fourth of July, and ethnic specialty nights—like Chinese or pizza—break up the scheduled menus discussed earlier. Socials are offered on a regular basis, sometimes associated with birthday celebrations or accompanying entertainment. As one resident says, *"There's always something going on in the afternoon."* Cake and ice cream, popcorn, sodas, or smoothies are served. ALs may also have socials serving wine and beer. At the Greenbriar, Ms. Washington comments that "each resident can get two glasses of wine but with the ice there isn't very much wine in the glass." That would still be fine for Mr. Braskey at Wetherby Place who laments that alcoholic beverages are not allowed: *"Can't even have any in your room."*

Besides food at meals and socials, ALs offer snacks at activities and sometimes in the evenings. The times they are available may not be optimal for the resident. For example, supper is served relatively early, averaging 5 p.m., and to accommodate an early dinner hour and time when staff is least busy, residents are offered snacks around 7 p.m. But 8 p.m. to 8 a.m. is a long time for some to be without food; consequently, residents tell us that they pick up something to eat later on before bed or while watching TV. At Winter Hills, Chrissy, a staff member, explained that residents were eating lunch and had the afternoon snack, and then were passing on dinner and, consequently, were losing weight. The AL had had a snack program that offered pretzels and cookies,

but now we do things like ham salad sandwich , like a half [of a sandwich] or cream cheese and cottage cheese, things that are more nutritional, so a lot them have gained their weight back, and I think it's more appealing than just dried up pretzels.

Most places do provide something on demand for a hungry resident, though it may be nothing larger than a packet of graham crackers. At other places, there is a "café" where residents know that fruit, beverages, and cookies are always available. For example, St. Brigid has a hospitality nook where "they have coffee and usually little treats and soda-fountain style chairs and round tables," according to one family member. What may be unusual is that at St. Brigid "there is a locked piggy bank out that suggests leaving a donation."

Importantly, residents' needs are met, if not by the home then by family members or by the residents themselves. Ms. Brubaker stated,

I always keep something in the little fridge there [in her room], and then I got me a jar of peanut butter over there and some crackers, so if I get real hungry at night I will bring some [thing] like sherbet, or sugarless ice cream and put it in the refrigerator and if I get hungry before I go to bed, I'll eat that. But I don't never go to bed hungry.

Families are very obliging. A retired military man, Mr. Reichelson, gets soups and chopped liver from his daughter to keep in his "locker." Ms. Pollock's daughter regularly brings by groceries.

Ms. Pollock: *[I] like frozen foods or canned things that I can dump out and warm up in there [microwave]. I've got little things—like carrots,...and a lot of little fruits. Those are great to open up—and puddings and all that.*

Researcher: And do you make—sometimes—a frozen dinner.

Ms. Pollock: *Yeah, and sometimes...They have at the store so many things you know—macaroni and cheese, you just pull the cover off and put it in—or things like that....[A]lso another nice thing my daughter does for me is hard-boil some eggs, I say don't bring many, and she might bring three and I can make egg salad, or I can slice them up and eat them for breakfast and I always have pineapple juice, or cranberry juice in there. I'm very lucky—I'm not complaining.*

Other options are for family members to carry in take-out food. Ms. Washington asked her son

to bake a potato for me. Or sometimes he'll bring one from Wendy's. Like he'll bring me hamburgers and a softie. Or he'll bring me something from Kentucky Fried [Chicken]. He won't get anything from Popeye's—I like their baked beans and rice and their chicken, it's spicy. And Burger King—I like Burger King.

As we read earlier in the book, Mr. Dugan's daughter Kathy considers herself a grocery delivery service for both her father and the staff he feeds in his room.

Kathy: I'm here probably two to three days a week for anywhere from 20 minutes to an hour...generally bringing groceries and unpacking them [24 cans of soda plus ice cream]....his generosity again. [Mr. Dugan doesn't drink soda.]

Researcher: What do you bring for him?

Kathy: I bring him some sort of deli meat—roast beef, corned beef....Bacon. Oh believe me none of these are heart healthy. But I've learned to pick and choose my battles; cream cheese, occasionally cookies, cashews—what [ever] else is generally on his list—orange juice....Or dried beef—you know, hot dogs.

But for residents without an outside support system, such as a family member, friend, or a volunteer from church, and especially for those whose own mobility is compromised, eating beyond the dining room is problematic.

DINING COLLECTIVELY

The Place

The dining room is the central space in the community life of an AL, and it is impossible to write about food without also considering place, people, and social interaction. The dining room is where residents gather and converse; it is one place where they are nurtured; and it is the public face that outwardly reflects the identity of the home. In some AL settings we studied, the dining room has the aura of an upscale hotel restaurant, with linen tablecloths, fresh flowers, and glass water goblets on every table. In other places, the dining area is an oversized extension of the kitchen, a large family room with paper napkins, seasonings, and bottles of ketchup and mustard atop easy-to-clean laminate-surfaced tables. On an early visit to the field site, the ethnographer wrote about Boxwood Gardens.

> I ventured into the dining room. Three staff members were changing tablecloths, green linen on top of white, and replacing artificial flowers and holders of creamers. There are about 14 round tables, seating 6–8 residents, and a few small tables for 2 and 4. Although the dining room is quite large, with one wall facing the small back yard composed almost entirely of windows, there is insufficient space for all the residents in wheelchairs to fit comfortably at one time in the dining room. (The tables are comfortably spaced for wheelchairs, which helps explain the need to have two seatings for meals.) Between the kitchen door and the dining room is a small pantry with soda and coffee machines.

None of the residents at Boxwood Gardens complained about the décor of the dining room; they especially appreciated the view of evergreens and sunlight streaming into the room from the glass wall. In another site, however, the researcher's description of the dining room was focused on its rudimentary physical appearance, whereas a family member considered this appearance to be a positive characteristic of the atmosphere of the AL. In fieldnotes, we read how the ethnographer is surprised by the medicalized nature of the dining setting of St. Brigid.

> There are windows flanking either side of this large room, lending the room lots of light. Probably the most distinguishing feature of the entire unit is its floors—shiny, well-maintained linoleum squares—very industrial-looking. It gives the place a very clinical and nursing home feeling, overtaking any of the other features that might give the feeling of something other than a nursing home.

This same researcher interviewed the daughter of a resident living there, who felt her mother's successful adjustment to St. Brigid was, in part, the result of her mealtime experience.

> The eating areas were just—I was very impressed with the dining rooms, because of the small tables, the assigned seating, but it's like a home atmosphere. The fireplace there, and the mantel and all the open windows, it just had an air of welcoming and comfort. You just felt like, you know you weren't entrapped in some little dark area.

Whatever its physical characteristics, and however the ambience speaks to a resident's preference, the dining room is the hub of social life, and often of health care, in AL settings.

As the hub of life in the home, eating brings everyone—residents, servers, and staff—together in sickness and in health, in good moods and bad, in one place two or three times daily. Residents who have been sharing meals with a partner or eating alone for a number of years find themselves in an often busy, somewhat chaotic and noisy place. Residents are walking or walkering in, propelling wheelchairs or driving their scooters, calling out to one another, sometimes stopping to check in with a friend before settling at their seats, which are often assigned by the staff. Servers are clanking plates and silverware, others are taking dinner orders. Staff yell across the room to each other, and if they happen to be from the same African country, may use the language indigenous to Sierra Leone or Nigeria. Polite conversations, jovial banter, and arguments occur, just like in any large family gathering, except that these residents are not family and most are not used to collective living. The senses are overwhelmed. There are smells of fish and beef, antibacterial cleaners and air fresheners, body odor and body lotion, all at the same time. The sounds are of voices, hushed and high-pitched, melodic and strained, nonsensical and lyrical, with sights of smiling and weary faces, upright posture and drooling chins. One can be touched by canes or brushed by fingertips. The tastes include food not routinely found at home. It takes time for adjustment.

The dining room is where collective living happens. Residents are nourished and intake monitored, reports sent to families and nurses on staff. Medications are administered with little concern for privacy. Residents keep up to date with each others' families and ailments. It is the quintessential communal experience, where the value of socialization, imbued in AL philosophy is expressed. Staff and administrators often value socializing in this environment so highly that in some ALs, residents are penalized if meals are delivered and consumed alone in their rooms. The few who are fit and able but refuse to come to the dining room are charged a stiff fee for the room tray. When the fees appear on a monthly statement, optional meals in one's room may become an issue with residents' children as well; the children may also actively encourage eating in the dining room, even for a parent who is a self-professed "loner." Money trumps privacy.

Significantly, we found, overwhelmingly, that residents may not like what is served but they enjoy going to the dining room. They congregate near its door, visiting or waiting silently, some lining up an hour before a meal, waiting for the okay to walk in and take their places. Residents meet up with tablemates, and for some residents, these are the only people they know well at all, in the AL. Ms. Rawlings of Wetherby Place confided that "I stay to myself....I don't know a lot of people." The dining room gives her an opportunity to socialize. "I know the people I eat with at every meal. They're very very nice. I like them." But, as the story of the three men at the Greenbriar in Chapter 2 showed, assigned tablemates sometimes are warmly congenial and other times may be simply tolerant of one another's presence, habits, and foibles.

Residents use the dining room to talk to others. We found that residents don't visit each other in their rooms, as a rule, but prefer instead to interact in public spaces. Beside attending activities, taking naps, meeting appointments, and getting "stuff" done, residents find the dining room to be the perfect venue to exchange ideas and gossip. Residents gripe about the food, share the latest things on the news and family or just talk about just things in general. They may converse about everyone liking the food, that's one good topic, sports, or the weather, their children, how old they're going to be, what they want to do, who died and who's where...which aide is coming in and which is not. In other words, residents talk about what everyone else does—not just about the past or ailments or problems, but what Ms. Gentile calls "chitchat."

> **Researcher:** What sorts of things do residents talk about when they get together?
>
> **Ms. Gentile:** *A lot of them bitch. [laughs] That's the only word I can think of. Or, gossip—"Did you know—did you know this, did you know that?" Or we talk about other residents that we know are ill or have gone to nursing homes or the hospital, "How is she or he?"—or whatever. That type of chitchat.*

It is also important to note that some residents say their tables are quiet; no one is talking. Although Ms. Rawlings likes the people at her table, "We don't talk too much....I'm glad." At Arcadia Springs, Ms. Burbridge observes that residents at other tables are talking, "but I have a table that they just don't [talk]." Family members were especially concerned about the lack of conversation. At Murray Ridge, Dee, the daughter of a resident suggested a television or piped-in music to enliven the dining room.

> *Researcher:*…people don't do a lot of talking?
>
> *Dee:* No. [pause] When we go down there, we try and go down at lunch-time so we could have lunch with her at the table and I mean we're the only ones doing any talking, our table. Because we involve everybody at the table in conversation and—
>
> *Researcher:* So why do you think that is?
>
> *Dee:* I don't know. Well a lot of them are not [exhaled breath]—a lot of them are a little "Alzheimery," [laughs] and they just kind of keep to themselves. And, you know, maybe if they had some just visual or mental stimulation it would [pause] start some conversation, I don't know.

Besides dementia and personality affecting the level of conversation, there is also compatibility. Sister Barbara at St. Brigid speaks succinctly to this point.

> The mealtime experience—you might have someone that's compatible at the table. It's very difficult for the residents when they have—are sitting with someone that's difficult. And sometimes in our unit there isn't too many places—any more openings. So sometimes residents are placed with people who they would rather not [be with].

Sister Barbara is referring to the assigned seating rule, an organizational tool often used in AL. It is an important structural component of the soft institution (see chapters 2 and 6).

The Soft Institution Revisited: A Microcosm of Food and Dining

The dining room exemplifies what we mean by a soft institution (see Chapter 2). There is a bureaucratic structuring of roles as well as a complex set of rules that reflect management policies and the philosophy of the setting. Care aides and dining staff moderate the meals and the residents' behavior. To help them accomplish this goal, they implement a policy of structured, orderly seating. We found that most ALs assign residents to seats.

"Does that work out OK?" an ethnographer asks Ms. Burbridge, a resident at Arcadia Springs. "Yeah, it seems like it. I would say the average person seems to be all right about it." Katey, a staff member, explains the reasoning at Winter Hills.

> *Katey:* They have assigned seating in the dining room and that's what they [the residents] request because they were tired of running in and saving—you know grabbing a table and saving it for their buddies. So we went around and asked everyone, alright who do you want to sit with, where do you want to sit—it's not written in stone, [laughter] because there are some days when they'll come and say oh, I don't want to sit with her anymore, I can't stand her table manners or, you know. We can almost tell when somebody is moving in, who to pair them with to start off with in the dining room, because you can see different personalities and how well they get along.
>
> *Researcher:* So if somebody wants to move, if somebody comes down to dinner tonight and says, I don't want to sit there any more—
>
> *Katey:* Then they can move.
>
> *Researcher:* Right away they can move.
>
> *Katey:* If there is a place right away, otherwise we'll work with them and work around and see if we can get someone else to trade. It might not happen that day, but if there's an empty seat, it can.
>
> *Researcher:* That would be—I wonder if the other residents would know—this woman is leaving my table because—
>
> *Katey:* They do know, they do know. But at that—it's funny, because I don't know what it is, they talk real loud about each other. [laughs] They're aware.

ALs assign seats for efficiency and convenience. What is interesting is that once residents are assigned a seat, there is relatively little movement. Rather than being due to complacency or resignation, this is likely the result of the AL coordinator getting a good sense of a resident's personality and placing that individual with others having a similar nature and interests. What is even more interesting is that, in

ALs where residents choose their own seats, they rarely change them. Ms. Gentile describes her experience at her dining table.

Once you sit at a table it seems like those that are there expect you to be there. You know, that type of thing. And it's very rare that you don't sit at the same table. You might not sit in this seat, you might sit in this seat [pointing]...but usually you sit at the same table.

Sitting in one spot becomes ritualized; it is patterned behavior that helps individuals adjust to a collective dining experience (Frankowski, Roth, Eckert, & Harris-Wallace, 2011). A resident at the Greenbriar tells us that he sits in the same seat every day. "It's a habit." Another says, "I haven't seen anybody move. My friends eat at the same place." Residents, like most of us, are creatures of habit, and staking out a place, even when assigned, is comfortable. For Ms. Ames, who did change her seat at the Greenbriar to sit by herself, convenience was crucial in light of her health and mobility limitations.

When I first came here, I sat two or three other places before I ended up where I'm sitting now, because this spot seems to be the best. It's best for when I'm coming in or leaving the dining room as far as having enough space to maneuver and get around and not get in other people's way also. And the other reason, like I said, because I'm spastic and I'm still pretty active in my legs...it's really not set up [for people with leg problems]; it's more like...going to a restaurant.

Despite what Ms. Meisel, a resident at Boxwood Gardens, says, that once you have a seat at a table, "you're more or less stuck," residents can shift if they request a move to another table, like Ms. Ames did. To complicate matters, a full census [every room is filled] sometimes results in multiple seatings, where lunch and dinner are offered twice each per day. Meals are served at set times at the discretion of the dietary services coordinator, whose need to "go home" supersedes the residents' requests for eating later. But, as we have discussed previously, residents have the option to dine out (provided they have transportation) or buy their own groceries and eat prepared meals and snacks in their rooms at their leisure. Many ALs have rooms or suites that are equipped with microwaves and refrigerators, enabling some degree of autonomy for those preferring an alternative entrée or meal schedule—an option of particular importance to late sleepers. In addition, residents have asked for—and so far have been denied—ALs that have full kitchens where they could cook their own meals.

Institutional rules extend beyond scheduling. As we saw at the Greenbriar, residents are not permitted to take food out of the dining room and back to their rooms, which does not preclude residents from hiding leftovers on their person or in walkers. Temperatures of the food and diets are somewhat regulated; some complain that soup is never hot enough and the lack of seasonings reflects a standard low-salt diet. However, residents have the freedom to eat what they like. Cost affects what is purchased, resulting in the much-served canned peaches.

In other words, soft institutions allow maneuverability around a set of formal rules. What is important is that the structure adjusts to its personnel, consumers, and finances. If the setting is to be successful, it needs to be filled with contented residents. AL settings are not total institutions that operate under strict rules for its inhabitants, like prisons. Soft institutions allow for fluidity and change, and know they must attract and appeal to their resident base so they do not lose residents and go out of business.

Making Choices in the Setting

AL providers sometimes point to the dining experience as one daily arena for residents to exert choice by selecting their food preferences at any given meal—of course, from the menu options planned and presented by the setting's cook, chef, or dietary director/contractor. Residents are guided to choose what is best for their health, but they are also free to select what they want, irrespective of medical advice. Choosing by taste falls within the acceptable rubric of most settings; allowing residents to eat what they want and sometimes override prescribed medical diets separates AL senior housing from nursing homes and other skilled facilities, where the clear medical model constrains choices to those suitable for one's diagnoses and medical advice.

There were, of course, many opinions proffered in our interviews about the choices of foods, their preparation, and how well they were served (e.g., was the food already cold before it arrived at the table). While taste, of course, is relative, residents' preferences were often made very clear to us. "Whatever happened to plain cooking?" wondered

Ms. Gentile, who described herself as a "straight meat and potatoes" person. Ms. Carson, our number-one nutrition advocate, not surprisingly wants more greens; and, whereas Mr. Sterling needs more seasoning, other residents want none. We have learned that residents are all over the map with specifics and generalizations when it comes to taste, a situation that often confounds those attempting the impossible task of pleasing all of the people all of the time in terms of what foods to serve and how to prepare them. Tina, the Executive Director of Boxwood Gardens, shared her personal evaluation with us.

> Some of our residents, I mean they love junk food. They are junk
> food addicts. When we have…theme night…[the cook will] ask
> them—what do you want tonight?…Sometimes they pick Pizza,
> you know or they'll pick—…they wanted Chinese food one night,
> so we had egg rolls, and the soup, I'm thinking oh, my goodness—
> the sodium, their blood pressure is going to be sky high. But they
> enjoyed it, and they come up and they talk about it and they
> absolutely love it. And then I have some that you know—if it's not
> organic—we all are going to hell.

An interesting example comes from St. Brigid, when the cook tried to "spice up" their soups. This innovation didn't sit well with Ms. Bachman.

> *You don't get any noodles in the soup, you get…big bow tie things. Well,*
> *how are you supposed to eat those bow ties that come in the thing with the*
> *soup?…You'd have great big pasta—not noodles. I would eat the soup if*
> *it had skinny noodles in it you know, but you would get great big chunks*
> *of pasta, and to this day I won't eat no pasta.*

Another try at soup also didn't fare well with Ms. Bachman.

> *I mean, we never got food like that when we were kids…sometimes*
> *you'll have soup—it was supposed to be Italian Wedding soup. Well, I'm*
> *not Italian, I never heard of Italian Wedding soup and when I got it, it*
> *had—whoever made it must have took the leftover spinach and dumped it*
> *in the soup and you had to eat a lot of those spinach leaves.*

Despite the two soups' popularity in restaurants and supermarkets, Ms. Powell, another resident at St. Brigid, concurs in her opinion with her neighbor.

They got soups here I never even heard—onion soup, wedding soup—I said "Who likes that stuff?" Now they have beef vegetable soup—it was almost like black, and I said, who in the heck ever—put black soup on the [menu]—and I said just give me a half a dipper full and then I didn't eat it all. [W]hy don't they just make a decent kind of soup and a sandwich?

Whereas some residents want "decent" soups, others mention redundant choices on menus. Ms. Kates at Wetherby Place notes that

Their food is fine, but it's like I said—it's too much turkey, and chicken, and beef. And every time I look at the menu, turkey and beef—oh, forget it. They could make like macaroni and cheese, they don't always have to have meat on the menu, you know, you can have other things too. I'm bringing it up when we have a meeting. Oh, yes, I'm bringing it up, absolutely.

Ms. Kates hopes that her participation in Resident Council, a monthly meeting in which all residents can offer suggestions, accolades, and criticisms about collective life, will bring results. Dr. Luckinbill, a resident at Wetherby Place, has a more personal approach. He points out that residents with different backgrounds have different expectations, even of the same recipe. People aren't always willing to try something new, he commented. For him, menu redundancy turned out to be positive.

Researcher: What makes a meal good?

Dr. Luckinbill: Taste. Like, they'll have beef stroganoff today. Then we'll have chicken fricassee for lunch. Well, I'm not a picky eater, so beef stroganoff can be small tips of beef and some gravy spread over noodles. . . . As far as I'm concerned, that's right. But there may be a person here who looks at that and says that's not beef stroganoff, because it doesn't have this or it doesn't have that. They have an item, but see, items recur on this menu. And so, one item that recurs is a pizza, but it's a vegetarian's pizza and I shrugged it off the first couple of times, but one day I didn't like the alternative, whatever it was. So I tried it, they call it a veggie pizza, and it wasn't bad!

Researcher: So the meals most of the time. . . .

Dr. Luckinbill: We live from meal to meal. One of my tablemates is 100 years old. He never complains. We get weighed once a month. This pot belly—I've gained 50 pounds, so I stopped eating desserts.

Dr. Luckinbill did more than that. Upon taking on the job of Resident Council President, he planned to ask the chef to offer a 1,500-calorie option for every meal. "I used to be handsome," he moaned.

Although some express discontent, others appreciate the options served. At St. Brigid, Ms. Howard finds, "The food's quite good. I enjoy eating the food." The majority of residents in our sites would agree with Mr. Braun at Winter Hills, "It's not like a home-cooked meal, but for a second home it's the best you can do." Residents in AL do recognize that choices and options for how food is prepared are constrained by an institutional framework.

It is interesting to note that the main area where choice is honored, choices from the menu, has one of the greatest potential impacts on health. Rather than erring on the side of nutritious diets and encouraging residents to eat healthily, as advocated by Ms. Carson, care staff support the value of decision-making and acknowledge that residents have the right to make bad choices. Perhaps if more appealing healthy choices, such as quality sugar-free desserts, were encouraged and offered to diabetics, and more fresh fruit and less canned peaches were available, a growing number of residents would choose foods wisely.

The expression of power and control is also reflected in this social institution. The example of Ms. Carson asking for bananas, discussed earlier in the chapter, speaks to this control. Staff often disregard the residents' knowledge and use strategies such as refusing to hand over bananas to demonstrate their power over them. Donna, a staff member at Arcadia Springs, evaluates her coworkers.

> *Researcher:* I wanted to ask you about the dining room. You said something about people can get testy.
>
> *Donna:* Yeah, because there's a lot of people in a small area and when you have a lot of wheelchairs, they are getting clinked up with each other, you know, and then not to mention you have got staff in the dining room who aren't always pleasant.
>
> *Researcher:* The waitstaff?
>
> *Donna:* Right. And granted, some of the residents are demanding, but I feel like that's your job, so just deal with it. You know, stuff like that.
>
> *Researcher:* Like the customer is always right.
>
> *Donna:* Well, yeah—but sometimes they ask for little requests and the dining staff acts like it's a major ordeal. I don't know if that's

about power or what, so I think that—yeah that, it was not even just that. It's also like, you know, this little resident might be mad at this little resident who is sitting there, and, you know.

Researcher: Interpersonal stuff too. That's harder to control. But the idea of pleasant waitstaff, that's something that—

Donna: That's a big, big thing. Our waitstaff is not always very pleasant, and it bothers me.

Returning to Ms. Carson at Boxwood Gardens, the hierarchal attitude of staff over residents is present in this instance, despite the fact that the resident is ostensibly the consumer and has already paid for her fruit. Ms. Carson is forced to negotiate—or even beg—to take three bananas back to her suite, after proving that she knows the difference between a raw and ripe one! Residents who fail in, or opt out of, negotiation are left without their easily met preferences being addressed, or else they are made to spend more money to buy what they want, or have to rely upon others to buy it for them.

The dining room, then, is the most visible place where AL philosophy is publicly expressed and observed. Although having the ability to choose an entrée is sometimes equated with independence, albeit superficially, selecting food is important to residents and most go to the dining room regularly. The dining experience occupies a large percentage of time in a resident's day, and although choices are often not the most nutritious or palatable, residents find something among alternatives, wich leaves a few residents to exist on hot cereal or processed cheese and white bread sandwiches. The alternative is cereal or the sandwich. Residents choose what best approximates their diets before move-in, and staff monitor choices to make sure everyone is "adequately" fed. Unfortunately this oversight lends itself to a power differential, in which it is possible for staff to exert control over residents' decision-making.

FOOD AND DINING AS THE CRUX OF LIFE IN AL

Focusing on the Experiential Nature of Eating

Why are food and dining so important in AL? With all of their complexities, they comprise the center of everyday experience.

The dining room is where maximum social interaction occurs. People go and converse even when they don't like the food or aren't hungry. Eating provides an activity. It is something to do. It takes up time for three segments of the day. It structures daily life and provides stability in transitioning to senior housing. For some, it is the high point of the day. They see people, even if they don't talk to them. Many are happily reminded that they no longer have to cook, whereas others sadly recognize their loss of ability to make their favorite recipes. Some express their autonomy over their day in part by choosing their meals and overriding their doctor's concern about salt intake. Eating fills the gnawing hunger in their stomachs, sometimes with nutritious food, and hopefully with choices that taste good, and if they don't like it, they can sit, like the residents at Ms. Gentile's table, and "bitch" about how heavily they pay for this amenity.

The dining room signals to residents that they are members of a collective living setting, which some residents humorously call a "dormitory" with a "cafeteria." It provides a source of interaction, which is expected by the AL industry. Except in rare instances such as Ms. Ames's, there are no tables for one, thus underscoring a sense of camaraderie and communitas, reinforced by special events that take place in the dining room on holidays and birthdays.

The dining room also underscores differences between the residents, some more frail than others. It bothers Ms. Carson to see residents "when they're sick and can't feed themselves"; her daughter laughs that she'd go to the dining room more often if she could discuss "the theory of relativity or something like that!" One daughter talks about an encounter with her dad at Wetherby Place.

> Unfortunately, we got there right around dinner time, so everybody was kind of congested in the entry getting ready to go in—so we kind of—not have [had] to fight our way through people, but there were a lot of people and quite a few of them were in wheelchairs and his first look and first reaction was very negative, and he never overcame that, seeing people in wheelchairs. And that was really hard on him and I kept saying to him, their bodies are in wheelchairs, not their minds, talk to them, Dad. And my father, who had been this outgoing, [pause] wonderful person had changed... When he came he was friendlier; there were a few more active residents, you know, as

the population has changed and he had one really, really nice friend. Another gentleman was [of the] same background, and ate at the table with him, and liked different foods and they would sometimes get carryout and share it. New foods—my father was talking about—food is [of] primary importance to my father. It's really the thing that keeps him going, and that gentleman has died and since he has died, and that was a couple years ago, [my dad] has not really made another friend and he kind of is very resistant. [The social worker] said that that's a very common thing. People are afraid to make friendships because they lose those friends, you know, they're older; it's harder to make friendships.

Although it is not uncommon for residents to be uncomfortable with illness or dementia, it is more common to observe residents helping one another, exemplifying one type of friendship. Residents bring neighbors to dinner, cut up their food, and encourage eating. Ms. Ashman cares for a much older lady who she says has become "sort of a mother to me." Ms. Wyler of Boxwood Gardens invited a man to her table. "He looked so feeble and didn't know where to go....My problem is, when I see somebody who doesn't know what or where or—somebody new—and I have a place, I take them on." Others encourage friends to eat. Ms. Gentile found an acquaintance at Boxwood Gardens from her old neighborhood, who was displaying increased dementia. She comments:

> She has trouble remembering and she forgets why she's in the dining room—you have to remind her to eat—eat.... She's sitting near me. I go "Nellie, eat your sandwich," or "eat your cereal" or "eat your dinner." I remind her.

For the AL owners, the dining room is the image of their identity. It is a place highlighted on tours by marketing directors, and potential clients are encouraged to partake in meals and conversation before signing their contracts. For the administrative staff, food and eating serve as a way to organize daily experiences. It reflects the census [number of residents], and must accommodate more or fewer residents with variations in budgets by numbers of seatings and menu options. It is where cultural practices are noticed. It is also the place where the AL and its staff exercise their power by enforcing rules (seatings, style of serving) and by their oversight, as will be discussed in more detail in Chapter 5. Staff are generally highly supportive; they can also be demeaning and controlling.

Challenges to AL Dining

ALs are regulated and tasked with providing food as a personal care service. This involves making sure that residents eat or are being fed in compliance with their individualized care plan of activities of daily living. Within the state of Maryland, this includes the provisions that each resident be given three meals daily in a common dining area with additional snacks available 24/7; that meals be "well-balanced, varied, palatable, properly prepared, and of sufficient quality and quantity to meet the nutritional needs of each resident with specific attention given to the preferences and needs of each resident"; that food preparation adhere to state and local standards for safety; that menus be provided with advance notice and kept on file in the home; that special diets be prescribed and recorded; and that residents be monitored (Maryland regulations). Essentially, what is mandated is decent and plentiful food, routinely provided under safe conditions.

This can be a tall order for ALs where their interpretation of the regulations often differs significantly from that of the residents, and where the implementation of the regulations is affected by philosophy, budget, census (the number of residents living in the AL at any one time), and capability and efficiency of staff. Food and dining present significant challenges to both management and residents in AL settings. The home is faced with residents of a variety of backgrounds, tastes, needs, and expectations, to which they must provide services determined by regulations, AL goals, individualized care plans, income disparities, cost, and staff fluctuation. To complicate matters, there is much subjective interpretation as to the meaning of "well-balanced, varied, palatable, properly prepared...[and] sufficient quality and quantity" to meet each resident's daily nutritional needs and preferences. Whether it is the lack of "meat and potatoes" or "leafy and green vegetables," Boxwood Gardens and every other AL has to address the interpretation of the regulations for their residents.

It is challenging to prepare food that residents like within the AL budget, and there are generational, regional, and ethnic differences to consider. Arguably, it is reasonable to expect that not all meals will be appreciated by all residents, and at Boxwood Gardens canned peaches became a symbol of all that is wrong with the food. Researchers attending Resident Council and Food Committee meetings record the variety in preferences: some residents demand crunchy vegetables, others request them soft; some residents ask for stewed meat, others favor roasted. Susannah, the daughter of Ms. Pollock in Boxwood Gardens, provides an insightful evaluation into the "generational palate" of her mother's cohort:

> All right, I actually think it would be easier to say what my mother doesn't like and I—how I perceive those dislikes. First of all my mother hates the food at Boxwood Gardens. She just—she finds it really bad. Now I've sat through enough meals with her there that I feel they have good days and bad days. And I do think that they put more care and effort into those meals where family members are likely to be present and that kind of irks me. So, I don't think the food is intolerable. I do think one problem with the food is that they do not fix the residents the food that the residents grew up eating, or ate in their own homes. They don't fix things like tuna-noodle casserole, they don't fix things like meat loaf and mashed potatoes and it can't be for economic reasons, I believe it must be because those foods are deemed too starchy or something, but those are the comfort foods that people of that age require.
>
> I mean the foods that they give them sometimes, it's hilarious on the day when they serve sandwich wraps for lunch, because every plate goes back with the wrap almost untouched. These people do not eat sandwich wraps. They're an alien food for them. My generation eats sandwich wraps, younger generation, so they [the AL menu planners] don't really pay very much attention I think to the food that would be comforting to the residents who live there.

Susannah suggests, then, that meals be tailored to age cohorts. She also addresses the business of food.

> They don't always have a muffin in the morning, for example, and I do know that because all of their food is prepared in one central location and trucked to the various Boxwood Gardens. There may be times when they are low on a certain commodity.

And that also means that the food that they prepare needs to be easily warmed up. Most things are swimming in gravy or sauces, which my mother detests, and which I don't think are healthy. I don't eat gravy, so while I don't think that it's as bad as my mother thinks it is, I think there are problems with the food. And even if there weren't problems with the food, if my mother detested the food, that would still be a problem. There is something they're not listening to if the residents don't like the food. And I hear many more complaints than from just my mother.

Comfort, regional, and generational foods need to be incorporated into the business of food. Liver and onions, scrapple, hot dogs and beans, macaroni and cheese, tuna-noodle casserole, and meat loaf and mashed potatoes are as important as leafy greens and brown bread.

It is also challenging to consider the needs and preferences of each individual resident when the group of them lives collectively within an institution (albeit soft) staffed by relatively few employees. Mr. Portoni spent hours each day attending to his mother in Boxwood Gardens when, because of his poor health and advancing age, he could no longer care for her in their home. He got to know the residents in her corridor well and often assisted in their care. He advises staff, "You need to expand your horizons here. These people are not vegetables," and describes the need of person-centered care in AL, including for those residents with dementia, an approach fostered by the Center for Excellence in Assisted Living (Love, 2010), with strong support from the Centers for Medicare and Medicaid Services (LaPorte, 2010). CMS's recent guidelines not only embrace, among other changes, the decorous dining rooms (served meals, china metal cutlery, tablecloths) offered by many ALs, but also suggest that ALs prohibit "staff interactions and communications only with each other rather than with residents while assisting them" (LaPorte, 2010)—actions we observed in our sites on a regular basis. Research data support Mr. Portoni, who espoused encouragement to residents (see Chapter 3), as this results in increased food intake and a more positive eating experience (LaPorte, 2010).

An environmental challenge to consider is the apparent disconnect between the restaurant model of the dining room in AL and the housing administrators' premise that the AL is home. Homes do not have restaurants, and AL for most is not quite home. Restaurants offer a multiplicity of choices, and choice is a value espoused by the AL philosophy; choice is, however, limited in each specific setting. Another difference is that the resident in the dining room has no redress if the menu option is not of expected quality, unlike in a restaurant, where the meal is sent back to the chef. Also, restaurants do not have assigned seats and are not concerned with compatibility of clients. AL kitchens are more like home pantries stocked with basics, offering few options for meals. If a restaurant is to remain in business, it needs efficiency and fast turnaround of customers. That isn't so in AL. Residents complain that, often, there is a long wait between the time their order is placed and when it is delivered to their tables. Space is also a factor, with residents lining up to wait for the dining room to open or for their assigned seating time, and this attracts complaints from other residents. In an interview, the researcher asked a resident what she would do differently if she were in charge of the functioning of her AL.

> *If I was in charge of this place the first thing I would do, I make sure that all these wheelchair patients stop blocking the aisles. They block the aisles—they all go into the dining room. And I would tell those patients I don't want you into the dining room until exactly 8:30—or 8 o'clock—we have breakfast at 8:30, not at 9:15 or 9 o'clock. They sit out there—then these wheelchairs are in everybody's way and I don't like that. And that's another thing that I would stop, is that brigade or that parade of wheelchairs. They have to park either in the hall by the walls, but they would not be allowed to park where they park, because they block every passageway. And I keep saying if there's a fire alarm or a fire what do you do with all these wheelchairs?*

The collective living–shared eating environment could benefit from a refashioning of what it purports to be—a source of nourishment for both body and soul—by examining attitude, space, expectations, product delivery, and levels of interaction.

Successes in AL Dining

Despite numerous challenges, there are many successes within the province of food and dining. Residents are getting sufficient food intake, one of the most common reasons for movement into AL. Because meals are provided, something they were unable to do on their own, and because they are encouraged to eat, residents become physically stronger (Eckert, Carder, Morgan, Frankowski, & Roth, 2009). Better health translates into a more active life—with residents participating in activities, going out with families and on field trips, and even taking vacations. Good health permits an increased number of individuals to age in place, thus eliminating their transition to nursing homes.

Also, the ambience of the dining room encourages social interaction, a core value of AL. The dining room provides a venue for individuals to meet, and the staff recognize the difficulty that many shy residents have in making even superficial friendships. We found, overwhelmingly, that residents enjoy going to scheduled mealtimes to socialize and get caught up on the local "news," even when they are not hungry or don't like the meal. Even "bitching" about the dinner has a positive effect on well-being, because one is conversing, strengthening social ties, and eating relatively healthy food. Ms. Morris, a resident at Boxwood Gardens, enjoys her table despite the food.

> *At my table we laugh so much, we just look like we're nuts. One woman at my table, Jeanette, she's a former nun, boy we have more fun. We laugh and people all sit there and ask why we have so much fun.*

Residents do enjoy socializing in the dining room. They tell us that "*I do enjoy going out there*"; it's "*when I get out and see people*"; and "*I look forward to getting out of my room.*" Ms. Rosenstein reminds us that "Meals are social. [Residents] like meals. Not only does it fill their belly, it fills their other needs." Furthermore, Michelle, a marketing director at Boxwood Gardens, notes that "I feel like food is something to bond over and they—that's when people come out of their shell. A lot of people stay in their room except for mealtime, so that's a chance for them to make friends."

In ascertaining quality within the domain of food and eating, nutritional, environmental, social, and physical attitudes need to be considered. This involves cultural space and time in which relationships among residents and staff are built and their social ties solidified. Beatrice, an African direct care staff at Greenbriar, points to the pleasure that both staff and residents receive from their dining room experience. "Most of them are looking forward to going to the dining room to chitchat with their friends. They talk; they play. Most of us, we are there just to sit down with them, playing and talking."

REFERENCES

Eckert, J. K., Carder, P. C., Morgan, L. A., Frankowski, A. C., & Roth, E. G. (2009). *Inside assisted living: A search for home.* Baltimore, MD: Johns Hopkins University Press.

Federal Interagency Forum on Aging-Related Statistics. (2010). Older Americans 2010: Key indicators of well-being. Retrieved from http://www.agingstats.gov/agingstatsdotnet/Main_Site/Data/2010_Documents/Docs/OA_2010.pdf

Frankowski, A. C., Roth, E. G., Eckert, J. K., & Harris-Wallace, B. (in press). The dining room as locus of ritual in assisted living. *The Gerontologist, 51*(4).

LaPorte, M. (2010). Providers revamp dining to please the palette. *Provider, 36*(8), 26–30.

Love, K. (2010). *Person-centered care in assisted living: An informational guide.* Washington, DC: Center for Excellence in Assisted Living.

Maryland regulations. Retrieved January 20, 2011, from http://www.dsd.state,md.us/comar/comarhtml/10/10.07.14.28.htm

5

Autonomy in Assisted Living

ORIENTING POINTS

- Autonomy and choice are central to residents' quality of life.
- Autonomy as it is expressed in assisted living can be enhanced by the "little things."
- Residents' reactions to constraints on their autonomy vary.

BACKGROUND

When the idea of assisted living (AL) was first conceived, it was in response to the more restrictive and carefully controlled environment of nursing homes. One of the goals of the AL movement was to encourage greater resident autonomy by offering more privacy and freedom of choice. The health needs of AL residents have increased since those early years, and so too have the demands on the AL to ensure an adequate, high level of care. As we discussed in Chapter 2, AL is in many ways an institution, though one with fewer regulations and restrictions than its counterpart, the nursing home. Diminished autonomy and control are key characteristics of an institution, even a "soft institution." Over the years tension has developed, pitting the AL values of autonomy and privacy against the expectations and demands on AL to provide a safe and healthy living environment.

A preponderance of residents take issue with some of the inherent restrictions of living in an AL, although we also heard from residents who appreciate these restrictions because of the counterbalancing oversight and safety AL provides. So, although we found variation in how people regard the importance of independence and autonomy, the AL's core value and the residents' desire is to preserve as much autonomy for residents as possible.

In this chapter, we first address the ways in which AL enhances autonomy; second, we develop some of the ways in which AL constrains autonomy, discussing aspects of life in AL that are consistently contested across settings; and third, we explore how self-determination is affected by ageism and the prevalence of dementia within AL. Next, we identify patterns of resident responses to the limits placed on their autonomy within AL. Finally, we consider the significance of what may seem insignificant and the effect it has on the balance of quality in AL from the resident perspective. We have found that the concept of autonomy, a culturally defined notion, is best understood, when adapted to this context, to reflect what bioethics philosopher George Agich refers to as *actual* autonomy (Agich, 2003). We illustrate how autonomy is often expressed in more subtle and less obvious ways in the long-term care context.

"They Won't Let Me Do Nothing"

Ms. Powell, a spirited 95-year-old widow, is especially vocal about her dislike of the restrictions at St. Brigid, finding herself at odds with some of the rules.

> ...*they won't let me do nothing.*...*I couldn't bring my own bed. And I turn around and I said, "Why can't I have my own bed?" She said, "You need a hospital bed in case you get sick, we can wind you up." I said, "I don't know who died in this bed!"*

She wished for a lock on her door, so when she leaves overnight she could be assured her things were safe, and for the freedom to clean her own room and make her own bed, if she wanted.

Past life experience certainly shapes the expectations that Ms. Powell and others bring into later life, and influences how they react to the restrictions on autonomy that come with living in AL or in any collective setting. Some people never learned to drive and were dependent either on family and friends or on public transportation to get around. Others may have grown up within a cultural subgroup with a communal approach to living space. Ms. Powell, however, was accustomed to fending for herself. One of 12 children from an immigrant family, she raised her children in a poor, working-class urban neighborhood. She characterizes herself as a fighter, speaking here about her resolve to never allow anyone to hurt her.

I could always do for myself, you know. Sometimes [my husband would] get real mad at me and, oh, if he hit me, I'd have killed him. I seen my father hit my mother. I said, "No man ain't going to hit me, because I would kill him." Oh, I take care of myself.

It is not surprising that Ms. Powell's response to life in AL would be to resist any impingement on her independence.

Although Ms. Powell expresses a strong negative reaction to the loss of her privacy and autonomy within her new living environment, it was her decision to move into this AL. She has found ways to work around some of those elements of daily life that she has most resisted—for example, she tidies her room and makes her bed before the housekeeper comes by in the morning. With no lock for her door, she places a piece of tape across the door jamb when she leaves for the day to inform her if anyone has been in her room while she was gone.

Decisions made by older adults that may appear to abdicate or relinquish control can, in fact, represent an exercise of agency, a good example of "actual autonomy." For some individuals we interviewed, the shift from total self-reliance to a setting with care is both a choice and a relief. A burden is lifted for the individual who has struggled to prepare meals, shop for groceries, and keep medications straight. Those who made an active decision to move into AL, like Ms. Powell, tended to also be those who were more accommodating and accepting of the constraints that come with their new collective living environment.

Before we examine in more depth the ways ALs restrict residents' autonomy, we turn to the ways residents expressed an increased sense of independence and autonomy by moving into AL. As we wrote in Chapter 1, what may contribute to this feeling of increased autonomy is often a result of a comparison that is being made—either with where they had lived before or with the alternatives that may have been considered.

ENHANCING AUTONOMY

In many circumstances, a person's health may improve once he or she has moved into an AL. Services such as oversight of medications, regular nutritious meals, and regular monitoring of blood pressure and blood sugar, for example, can make a resident feel better. Reduction of the physical demands in one's home setting, such as climbing steps, getting and preparing food, and negotiating personal care and household tasks may also play a part, as the following dialogue shows.

> *Mr. Guarino:* I wasn't eating.
>
> *Researcher:* Really?
>
> *Mr. Guarino:* So to speak—pretty much—certainly not properly. I never ate breakfast or lunch. And I had somebody coming in every evening and they'd fix me a can of soup or something in the microwave or something. That was it. That went on for a couple months, maybe about three months. And boy, I said, I just can't—I've got to do something here. This is—because it was just getting worse. I'm walking better now [since living in AL].

Increased physical well-being enhances quality of daily life, perhaps providing a counterpoint to some of the more difficult aspects of a move to AL. Moving into a setting designed to facilitate greater mobility, with its elevators, widened doorways, and grab bars, also makes it easier to get around on one's own. Dr. Smith, an AL resident interviewed for a previous study, identifies the benefit of going from a split level home to an AL.

> One [bathroom] was up stairs, and one was down stairs, so for me to go to the bathroom I had to either climb, I had to negotiate the steps one way or the other. And that's one thing I don't have to face being here. They have an elevator that takes me up and down. And of course there's a bathroom right there.

Once the weight of keeping a home running—cooking, shopping, cleaning, and managing one's own medications—is lifted, residents often report a sense of relief. Only a few people told us that they missed tasks such as preparing daily meals. With the assistance received for daily activities, there is potentially more time and energy to pursue interests and hobbies, to rest, and to attend AL-provided activities (Hyer & Intrieri, 2007).

Some residents even appreciate the restrictions on coming and going from the AL. Ms. Wyler understands and recognizes the danger she could face being on her own outside of the safety of the AL. When asked if she ever goes beyond the sidewalk, she answered,

Oh, no. They [the AL] don't want you to go out on the main road.
They don't want you to go outside the gate. And I can see that, too.
People with wheelchairs shouldn't be out; if they fall in the street. And
then some people ... wouldn't know how to get back here if they got out.
They wouldn't know where they are, you know? So they don't—no,
they don't want anybody to go outside—unless you're going with
somebody. You sign out and then, unless you're going to a friend's
house or going shopping or to the doctor's, but you're always with
somebody.
... but most people wouldn't want to go out on the street on their
own, because it's too dangerous. ... I don't think many people want to
walk outside. There's plenty of room here to walk all around—front and
back and it's secure, at least, in here.

Beyond the physical dimension of care, AL can also fulfill an important social need. Before moving to AL, many older adults are socially and physically isolated, particularly if they experience health limitations. It may be the case for some that remaining in one's home may result in "dwindling choices and mounting levels of loneliness, helplessness, and boredom" (Thomas & Blanchard, 2009). Although some ALs offer more planned activities than others, living in such a collective environment provides an opportunity for increased social interaction for those who seek it. Before moving to Arcadia Springs, Mr. Guarino lived alone and really craved human interaction.

Researcher: You said you were living on your own for a while and it was too difficult?

Mr. Guarino: Much too difficult. I just can't—I let myself—I needed
companionship bad. Social interaction of any kind.

Researcher: Were you not getting out at all when you were—

Mr. Guarino: No, I couldn't. I couldn't. The doctor didn't want me to
drive. I lost a lot of the feeling in my hands. I knew I wasn't reacting
properly. I knew it—and I just couldn't drive; I couldn't use public
transportation.

By moving to AL, Mr. Guarino found a ready-made group of people with whom he could interact and socialize.

However, some people who seek greater social interaction may be disappointed to discover that many residents suffer from cognitive impairment. Those without cognitive impairment report experiencing difficulty finding residents with whom they can socialize. Mr. Guarino, a relatively young man of 62, found this to be true of Arcadia Springs, but had been prepared for this possibility.

> **Mr. Guarino:** *There aren't many around here that have all their marbles. They [the staff] tell me I'm the closest thing to someone that's sane.*
>
> **Researcher:** How does [knowing] that affect your interactions or your life here?
>
> **Mr. Guarino:** *I've got to fit in. This is something I knew coming here. The Department of Aging—they informed me very well—that all these people, that any place I went, people are much older and senile. They told me that. I knew that. I knew it's something I had to adjust to. And I have. I make sure—I go to everything.*
>
> **Researcher:** The activities?
>
> **Guarino:** *Yes. I go to everything here.*
>
> **Researcher:** Why do you do that?
>
> **Guarino:** *Social interaction—I like it.*
>
> **Researcher:** Even if some people you can't have a conversation with?
>
> **Guarino:** *Right, I still do. I just do it at their level.*

Residents like Mr. Guarino report developing friendships with staff members, because they have had difficulty developing mutually beneficial friendships with residents. For Mr. Guarino, his relationships with the staff are perhaps a more important part of his daily social life than his interactions with other residents.

> **Mr. Guarino:** *I use the staff a lot.*
>
> **Researcher:** For...
>
> **Guarino:** *Social interaction. They seem to accept me. I know that the other residents like me and the staff likes me too, I know that. They tell me that all the time.*

Living in a social setting such as AL, Mr. Guarino was no longer reliant on others to come to him for socializing.

Ms. St. John experienced a sense of accomplishment as a resident of Boxwood Gardens. She lobbied successfully for a public transit bus stop in front of Boxwood Gardens and secured a donated piano for the setting by placing a notice in the local paper. She was recognized as an effective leader by her fellow residents and staff members.

For the first time—I mean we really accomplished something and it was because I kept at it—I mean. That's because I kept them to an agenda and [did] not let anyone get sidetracked. And yet in some ways, I guess maybe you'd call me bossy, but somebody's got to be the leader. I mean I am the spokesperson for everybody. I am the—I'm the one they look to do things, and even the help does, too.

Fear of becoming a "burden" to one's family, a common and well-documented response to aging, can be moderated to some extent by moving into an AL. A resident from a previous study told us she wanted to avoid relying too heavily on her middle son, because her oldest son was undergoing chemotherapy for brain cancer.

I had promised [my son] that, while my other son was sick, I would stay here to give them a little peace of mind. Because they can't worry about him and worry about me at the same time. And they all have responsible positions and it's hard. What are you going to do, right?

Andrea North spoke very openly about the relief she—and she believes her father—felt once he moved into Winter Hills.

Well, that's another thing about being in a facility of any kind; if really intimate things need to be done, I don't have to do it. They're there. If he had to go into diapers I wouldn't—he wouldn't have to be embarrassed by having me deal with it.

For some older adults, simply being in a place that gives their children peace of mind allows the parents to be more self-sufficient—they are not as dependent on their children for their bodily, medical, or social needs as they would be if they were still living in the community.

CONSTRAINTS ON AUTONOMY

Although the interviews indicated some of the ways in which AL increases a resident's autonomy, the majority of residents we interviewed expressed some complaints or concerns about the loss of autonomy. The following sections examine two commonly shared concerns: securing a private space of one's own and coming and going as one pleases. We follow this discussion with another contested area of autonomy in daily behaviors—the use of alcohol, cigarettes, and sugar.

"This Is My Room; I'm Paying for It"

There is a level of self-determination that is expected upon becoming an adult. Having control over one's own space—as it relates to who we allow in, how we decorate and furnish it, and what we choose to keep in those private, personal areas—is crucial to the feelings of autonomy and independence. AL necessarily limits how individuals experience their personal spaces as it provides oversight and daily cleaning, and ensures safety.

St. Brigid's practice of requiring a hospital bed for all AL residents' rooms meant that a married couple we interviewed would no longer be able to sleep together. Because of the small size of the two small rooms the Griers were to share, the two hospital beds would not fit side-by-side. The Griers, as well as their daughter, spoke about this constraint. Asking about her parents' adaptation to life in St. Brigid, Joan said, "I think that the hardest thing here—they don't sleep together. . . . [My mother] was real funny—it was like, 'We need to touch bum-bums.'"

As we discussed in Chapter 2, residents do not have full control over who comes into their rooms. There are other kinds of restrictions in terms of what residents can and cannot keep in their rooms beyond furniture. For example Mr. Jones, who faithfully reads the *Wall Street Journal* daily to follow stock activity, disliked having his papers regularly thrown out by the housekeeping staff before he finished reading them.

> *Listen to me—listen to me—this is my room. I'm paying for it. If I want it messed up, I mess it up. But they don't like it. They'll walk in and see it on the floor. [. . .] If I want it on the floor it's there for a reason.*

Another resident was bothered when the staff made demands about furnishings she wanted to keep in her room.

> ***Ms. Harding:*** *I was upset when Sister took my rocker out and told me I can't have any rugs and that's because she's worried about me falling.*

And so I said, well, I have to swallow my pride and go through—if she's worried about me falling you know—so I gave my rocker away to one of my sons and gave my rugs away to another one of my sons. And so, she said that I could have—in the bathroom I could have the kind of sticky on the bottom [rug]—you know.

Researcher: How do you feel about that decision?

Ms. Harding: *Well, at first I was a little disturbed, because I didn't think it was an obstacle to me. But you know, you trust the Lord, and because it's done in love…it's not done through meanness, you know? And we can't always have everything we want so…[trails off]*

In-house policies and practices, such as forbidding the use of throw rugs on residents' room floors or carefully controlling the temperature of hot tap water to avoid burns, demonstrate how ALs are working to prevent or minimize hazards. But from the resident's perspective, these policies and practices also mean being unable to take a comfortably hot shower or to decorate their rooms, or retain favorite possessions as they would prefer.

Coming and Going

Having the freedom to come and go as one pleases is another significant marker of autonomy and control identified by many AL residents. Decreased physical mobility already greatly hampers some residents' capacity to get around. Dr. Smith, a retired professor and an AL resident after a debilitating stroke, aptly expressed this commonly held desire.

You know what really gets to me? When I see, I sit outside and I smoke. And all these people are leaving the building and all clutching car keys. And they get in their cars, and that chokes me up. I'm insanely jealous of that. But I have my moments like that. I know it sounds silly.

One's own set of car keys is in many ways symbolic of adult autonomy. With it comes an independence that is unmatched in other ways. Ms. Chapman echoes Dr. Smith's comments.

Driving is the most important. Oh god, I miss that something frightful. I miss that terrible. When you get a notion to do something or go somewhere and you can't do it. "Where's my keys?" They're gone.

The researcher followed up by asking what happened that made her lose her car or license.

Oh, I have my license—I still have that. I could go out and buy a new car if I feel like it. If I felt I was responsible enough I would, but I'm not sure I've reached that point. But if I do, I might consider that. Andy, my son— "Please don't do it," he says, because it might be dangerous to yourself or to someone else. You have to pay attention to those things, too. I don't like the idea that I would be dangerous to anybody, because if I felt that was dangerous I would not drive—because I wouldn't do that to anybody. Suppose you hit a mother with a couple of kids or something—wouldn't that be horrible?

One man at Arcadia Springs, Mr. Goddin, was stopped by a vigilant staff member as he attempted to make the short walk to the nearby convenience store for snacks, a trip he had been making regularly without any objection. *"One time, I was up at the convenience store here and the damn nurse came running up there: 'You don't supposed to be up here by yourself?'"* He lamented that he feels *"hemmed in,"* noting, *"I can't go nowhere—only look at television."* Mr. Goddin's daughter, who had been giving her father money to use at the convenience store, agrees with the facility's recommendation when they explained that he was gaining too much weight and raising his blood sugar to harmful levels with his junk food habit. After breaking his hip, this trek became impossible for him. His daughter, concerned with his diet, says his inability to walk to the store is a "good thing." She continues to bring in snacks and items, but has tighter control over his snacking choices.

As an alternative to going out on your own, most ALs offer some scheduled outings. But the destinations are predetermined by staff and seldom allow for extra stops at an individual's request. Some vans used by ALs have a limited number of spaces for wheelchairs. So many residents look for other opportunities to shop or get out into the community on their own. Frequently, this mobility support is provided by family members or friends, or sometimes these kin or friends serve as "designated shoppers." There are a few rare individuals who continue to drive their own cars, although, as Ms. Carson discovered, driving is not necessarily encouraged or supported by staff efforts. According to fieldnotes from an informal discussion with her, staff assistance in loading her scooter into her vehicle, which she was promised before moving into Boxwood Gardens, was not always provided.

Ms. McCoy, a resident of Arcadia Springs, tells about the time she was chastised for leaving without signing herself out at the front desk. Whereas a majority of the residents living there have dementia, Ms. McCoy does not. *"I'm not used to being told what to do and all this crap. I'm just used to going, and doing, and doing, and doing. When I used to drive, I was always going somewhere. That was my nature."*

Another resident described the staff vigilance over coming and going as a *"kind of spy network."*

Not all ALs deal with coming and going in exactly the same way, but most have some mechanism by which they keep certain individuals, particularly those with advanced dementia, from leaving. Determining who should be restricted from freely leaving the grounds gets complicated, and is not at all clear-cut. Complicating this further, residents who are allowed to leave will sometimes take along others who are known to wander or become confused. In such cases, enforcing a rule or policy becomes difficult, making the situation even more confusing to those who enforce it and those who must abide by it. Michelle, Boxwood Garden's marketing director, describes what she does when a resident wants to walk away.

> If a resident wants to walk away... you chase them through the parking lot and you try to redirect them. Like you don't tackle them, you can't restrain them physically and you can't restrain them chemically so it's, "Oh, where you going? Oh, you're going home. Oh, OK well—" You either just sit there with them, or if you—even if means walking with them.

Gae, the lead receptionist at Boxwood Gardens, described the dilemma faced by AL staff in her interview. When asked, "Who decides whether a resident can or can't leave? Suppose a resident comes down in the morning and says, 'Gae, call me a cab,'" she replied,

> Okay, well, now—I know all my residents. So I know who has the dementia and who does not, and who is capable. If I am real concerned, I will go and talk to our executive director. She makes the final decision on everything in this building. And I have had

concerns and I've had to go in to talk to her, and then she will call family, because this is assisted living. We cannot stop them.

Staff members are left in charge of policing the doors, sometimes without clear policy. Without obvious guidance, staff members rely on their own judgment, leaving room for interpretation, inequity, and misunderstanding. When the staff confronts residents at the door or chases them across the parking lot, this may be enough to discourage those with clear cognition from leaving again. One way residents have been able to overcome this restriction is to have a family member or person with power of attorney (POA) give permission for the resident to leave. In this way, the AL is ostensibly absolved from fault, should something happen while the resident is out. We will discuss this practice, sometimes referred to as *negotiated risk agreements* or *risk waivers,* in more depth in Chapter 6.

Cigarettes, Alcohol, and Sugar

These items are controlled or managed in varied ways across settings. For those residents whose prior lives included cigarettes and alcohol, restrictions on their use can be distressing, and a challenge to their sense of freedom. Dr. Smith continued earlier habits by regularly ordering a carton of cigarettes and a 12-pack of beer from a nearby liquor store, which delivered for a fee.

> **Dr. Smith:** *But they [AL staff] intercepted them at the desk. And in order for me to get it, I had to beg from the concierge two cigarettes at a time.*
>
> **Researcher:** So somebody downstairs would take the cigarettes out of the bag?
>
> **Dr. Smith:** *Right. And the only thing I can think of is they're afraid I'm going to smoke in my room. And I've been here for more than a year and I've never smoked in my room. I've never even been tempted to smoke in my room.*

The beer is then placed in the kitchen and also rationed out to Dr. Smith by the staff.

> *I'm supposed to get three a day and it seems like I spend half my life tracking down somebody—...But a couple of gals, in recent times, just*

said, "The heck with it. What's the matter with just giving you the beer, and you can dole it out yourself?"

Dr. Luckinbill lives in Wetherby Place, a religiously affiliated setting opposed to alcohol. Although it was possible to order an alcoholic drink with his meal on the occasional facility-organized restaurant outings, he had become physically unable to transfer himself from his wheelchair to a seat on the AL bus.

> *I used to go on every trip, whether it was a restaurant trip, whether we went to Red Lobster; we enjoyed ourselves. I would have a Bloody Mary with each meal. It's something you could never do here. They don't believe in coffee, whiskey, or anything else worthwhile. My kids would never agree to bringing me a bottle of whiskey to keep here, to take out of as I want to. And I miss the booze.*

Ms. Volbrecht, a resident of Boxwood Gardens, feels at the mercy of her son for her cigarettes. According to her interview, he refuses to give her discretionary money for fear she will buy cigarettes. Instead, he purchases cigarettes, which are then doled out by staff—one at a time. When asked how she receives her cigarettes, Ms. Volbrecht says her son controls this: *"I get 6 a day. I get one at 6 o'clock [a.m.], one after breakfast, one after lunch, one at 3 o'clock, one after dinner and one at 7."* Some family members, who have had ongoing concerns about a parent's drinking or smoking, will take the move into AL as an opportunity to restrict access to these substances.

In addition to alcohol and cigarettes, sugar is often restricted, or at least strongly discouraged, for diabetics in AL. Staff members are daily faced with requests that they know are within the residents' rights, but are nonetheless not good for them. For example, if a diabetic resident requests a sugary dessert, Marie, a care aide at Greenbriar, says she tries to talk them out of it. "We talk to them," she said. "This is not good for you. We got Jell-O; we got canned fruit." If the resident insists, she will concede: "Okay, you can have it today, one day. But tomorrow, I'm not going to give it to you." Despite her words of warning, Marie acknowledged to the researcher, "If they want, we've got to give it to them." Marie understood that giving in to the request was her duty.

Giving over control of these "forbidden" pleasures is very difficult for some residents and also challenging for families to control. Family members have been known to "sneak" junk food into their relative despite dietary restrictions or the AL's expressed order to refrain. Actions taken in these areas by the AL sometimes conflict directly with the espoused AL values of independence and choice.

THE INFLUENCES OF AGEISM AND DEMENTIA ON AUTONOMY

In the course of our research, we have observed the pervasive influence ageism has on residents' autonomy within AL settings. The prevalence of dementia within the AL population is a compounding factor, affecting how staff and family treat and regard a resident, whether or not the person in question is cognitively impaired. In this section, we consider these influences, hear how residents experience them in their daily lives, and explore how staff, consciously or unconsciously, make determinations daily about a resident's capacity to make choices and act independently.

According to prior research (Morgan, Gruber-Baldini, & Magaziner, 2001; Zimmerman et al., 2005), more than half of those living in AL have some level of cognitive impairment. By default, residents are often treated as if they all have memory loss and are unable to make decisions. This can lead to the troubling practice of disregarding a resident's request or assertion of fact. For example, when personal items go missing, staff often dismiss the resident's claim of theft and assume the owners forgot where they placed the items. The following examples are all drawn from situations that involve residents who do not have significant cognitive impairment.

Ms. Wyler recognized the problematic task that ALs like Boxwood Gardens face in determining whose recall can be trusted. Here, she speaks about managing her own medications: *"I guess they don't think I'm able. But I think in a place—these places—they can't differentiate who can and who can't [manage their own medicine]."* The real difficulty for AL staff and management is in identifying the presence and level of cognitive impairment, because the progression of cognitive impairment changes the assumptions made about resident autonomy. The consensus of family, administrators, and onlooking residents is that safety trumps people's right to come and go as they please in cases where residents may not remember where they live. Navigating the gray area between those who are mildly confused to those clearly requiring oversight poses a challenge for providers and family members alike.

At times, staff will disregard something the resident is trying to tell them. Ms. Riggs of Arcadia Springs, for example, tried to explain to the aide helping her get dressed that the clothes she was putting on her were not her own.

> *...one morning the girl was dressing me and she put my bra on and...I said, "that feels tight—don't feel like my bra." She said, "Well, it can't be anybody else's." And I said to her—"well, I don't know, it don't feel right." So she come out here for something and, while she did, I lifted my blouse and I looked and it wasn't my bra. And I said to her—"I'm sorry hon, but this is not my bra." She said, "Oh, yes it is—it was in your drawer." I said, "It isn't my bra." She said, "Well, if you insist." So she took it off, and I said "I don't want anybody wearing my bras and I don't want anybody to have to wear mine."*

Some residents, like Ms. Pollock of Boxwood Gardens, described having to insist to the medication aide that the pills she was being handed were not correct.

> *I know what I take, and it happened to me twice. I said the first time, "These aren't my pills." "Oh yes, Ms. Pollock, they're your pills." I said, "Would you please do me a favor and just check it?" And she left, you know, and she said, "Oh, you're right, they aren't your pills." See if I—sometimes they say, "open up" to people—plop. I don't like that....And then the other time, it was—they had the right pills, but there was only three. And I said, "Where's my fourth one?" because I have to take a blood pressure pill in the morning and at night. And I have to have that or it will go sky high or I'll drop. They said, "No, you've got them all." I said, "No I don't." I had to insist this time, because it's the blood pressure pill. And they went through, and through, and through and found it in another drawer.*

In a dramatic reversal of roles, some residents' children, friends, or other close relatives have primary legal control and authority through power of attorney (POA) or simply hold decision-making power due to the processes of the AL. Some of the ALs make it a practice to communicate with the family members about important issues, rather than

directly with the resident. For example, some sites where we have conducted research insist that we notify family members and POAs to give
them the chance to refuse to have their relative interviewed. This refusal
took precedence, even if their relative wanted to participate and was not
suffering from cognitive impairment. Some ALs defer to the residents'
wishes if they assert themselves early on and continue to act independently. However, more often, families or the POAs tend to be involved in
most big decisions. Janet, the daughter-in-law of a resident at St. Brigid,
said when asked about her mother-in-law's wishes, "Sometimes, even
your [own] choice is not the *right* choice, or what *we think* is the right
choice." Janet acknowledged the irony of her remark with a laugh, understanding how freedom of choice operates differently in this context.

The preferences, attitudes, and beliefs of the family members have
an enormous influence over the resident's daily life, and it can be both
positive and negative. Family members leave instructions with the rec-
reation coordinators to get their relative involved in more activities,
even when the relative has made it clear that she prefers to be alone in
her room, reading. Janet again speaks about her mother-in-law and the
conversations she has had with the staff at St. Brigid:

> We've talked about it, you know—just drag her to church, you
> know. Make her go out. And when she does it, she has a good
> time. But, you know, she is less likely to opt herself to do that. And
> sometimes they do, and I understand it's an assisted living, it's not
> total. And, you know, you can't force somebody to do something,
> but, and they do try.

One daughter said, "I like the fact that he has to come down for at
least two meals. He has to get off his duff and come down."

To be fair, the impulse behind a family member's demands is the
desire to see their parents happy and socially engaged. There are also
those children who work very hard to preserve a parent's autonomy as
much as possible, given his or her cognitive or physical needs (Funk,
2010). When Nancy Wells got a call about an opening from the AL of
her mother's first choice, she was faced with another decision. Nancy
told her mother of the call, despite her mother's cognitive impairment
and that her mother was already settled in at Winter Hills.

> My mother said to me, "*Am I going?*" I said, "Well, do you want
> to?" She said, "*No.*" I said, "Well then, you're not." I said, "You're

not. If you wanted to move, we would certainly take a look at it together. But if you're happy—" and I'm thinking, "I don't want to go through another move." So it wasn't my first choice.

In addition to the influence of societal ageism and the prevalence of dementia, AL residents, because of their declining physical and/or mental health, tend to have fewer resources to maintain balanced relationships, including those with AL staff who are providing care. This change in relationships, whether inside or beyond the AL, presents a threat to the quality balance. The most tragic result of this imbalance is when residents feel they must "exchange compliance—the most costly of all generalized reinforcers—for their continued sustenance" (Dowd, 1975). Within AL, there is little opportunity to alter the imbalance of social relationships. One example of how this imbalance plays out in AL is the common rule that forbids residents to offer gifts or monetary tips to the staff. Ms. Jacobs explained how being unable to give a gift to a staff member's new baby made her feel. *"See, it takes the humanness out of it. I don't like that, but I don't know that I can do anything about it either. So I just go along with them."*

Ms. Heilbrun from Murray Ridge is keenly aware that her friendships have changed since moving to AL. Unhappy with the imbalance that she feels has developed in her relationships with outside friends since living in AL, she said in her interview,

> *I have nothing to talk about. I don't do anything with anybody and I have nothing. And the activities are not something I can talk about; there's just nothing. It's like living in a jail....I have a couple of friends at home, and two of them still come and visit me. But it's—they have their own lives. They're widowed. Their lives are not made pleasant by coming to visit me.*

From Ms. Heilbrun's perspective, AL has stripped her of her ability to meaningfully contribute in social contexts of which she was once a part. We discuss this dynamic later in this chapter, when we address a commonly held belief among residents and family members that failing to comply may result in retribution.

RESIDENTS' REACTIONS TO DIMINISHED CONTROL

The constraints on autonomy and control that one might encounter upon moving into AL may not be apparent initially. It is only after living in the setting for a period of time that residents begin to fully realize how they feel about, and react to, this new environment. Mr. Jones, a resident at Boxwood Gardens, spoke of this in his interview.

> *Well, I think that everybody's different—just like when you go to buy a house. You like something in that house. You're like, "what?" Like, the way the furniture is made, when you have to walk down the steps, whether you've got to do this or that. Wouldn't you do that if you were buying a house? Well, you don't know that in assisted living. You don't know until you come in here or unless you got a friend that's in here, and will the friend tell you what's really going on here?*

Most of the residents we interviewed recognize the inherent tension between receiving the help and oversight they need while still maintaining all of the freedoms to which they are accustomed.

The following section identifies four categories of resident responses to reduced autonomy. The four categories are (1) understanding, acceptance, and accommodation; (2) fear; (3) assertiveness; and (4) advocating for others who may be more vulnerable.

Understanding, Acceptance, and Accommodation

A common response from residents is to explain to themselves and others the reasons for any impingement on their autonomy. Residents rationalize and accept practices that limit their control in daily life. Ms. Marshall, a resident at Arcadia Springs, speaking here about some personal items she needs, is at once understanding and accepting.

> **Ms. Marshall:** *But they don't want me to walk up there [nearby convenience store]. I guess they are afraid. They think I might get sick or something. But my disease is under control. I don't have problems. They're doing it for their own safety, I can see. They're doing it for their own safety.*
>
> **Researcher:** *So what are you going to do?*
>
> **Ms. Marshall:** *I have to do what I'm told. So my daughter took me out to the dollar store today because I wanted to get some Kleenex.*

Although she disagrees with the restriction as it applies to her, she understands and accepts the AL's precautionary measure and has found a workable solution.

Whereas Ms. Marshall represents those who made a proactive decision to accept the restrictions in AL, others felt defeated. Several residents we interviewed expressed their dissatisfaction but felt powerless to change what they believed was beyond their control. Although critical in his interview, Mr. Leland of St. Brigid could not see a reason to pursue his complaints.

> *So you complain. Does that help? I don't think—maybe for the instant you complain. But will you get any action out of it? I don't think—just what I've seen again living here, you know.*

One mechanism residents use to share their complaints is to participate in the periodic Resident Council meetings. However, the Resident Councils were almost universally ineffective in terms of providing meaningful voice to effect change. Residents were reluctant to speak up in meetings. When no feedback was forthcoming, administrators could easily interpret the silence as a vote of approval. Based on our observations of these sessions, as soon as the administrators walked out of the room, the previously silent residents would begin to grumble and express concerns. When asked why these complaints are not expressed during the meetings, several residents cited examples of times they would bring a concern to the meeting, but there was no action or follow-up. The one topic in the Resident Council meeting setting for which almost everyone seemed comfortable offering complaints or advice was food. But some administrators intentionally steered residents away from food complaints, because it could be such a contentious and idiosyncratic topic.

Accepting a decreased sense of autonomy can be a powerful choice. Older adults may decide to abdicate certain responsibilities to an adult child, for example, or defer decisions to others, but this is not always an indication that they have given up their agency—in fact, it can be quite the opposite. Mr. Epworth, a resident of Arcadia Springs, was quick to recognize the need for help and was comfortable giving his sister-in-law control over his finances and medical decisions.

> *Mr. Epworth:* *She's my—what you call it?—anyone who takes care of everything?*
>
> *Researcher:* Power of attorney—does she have your [durable] power of attorney?

Mr. Epworth: Everything. Got the whole works.

Researcher: Was that a decision you made? Did you decide to give her the power of attorney?

Mr. Epworth: Oh, yes. I talked to a lawyer about it. I said, I can't drive—I can't drive my car. I've got a house—I can't go back to the house, can't walk up and down the steps, so I've got to turn it over to somebody. And she's good—I've known her since she was 14 years old.

Ms. Thompson of Murray Ridge could appreciate the wisdom of relying on younger relatives with more physical energy.

I have nephews and nieces that have done an awful lot for me, since I've been in this nursing home [sic]. I tell you—I don't know what I'd have done without them. Moving things back and forth, we have properties we're selling and bringing things here. . . . They have energy, more energy than you have when you grow old.

Some residents are quite adaptable and flexible. For example, during an interview that took place in Mr. Guarino's room, the researcher was taken aback by the room's extremely loud air conditioning unit.

Researcher: It's so quiet in here now [referring to the a/c, which just turned off]. It really makes a lot of noise.

Mr. Guarino: Yeah, it doesn't bother me anymore. It used to, but not anymore. When I first moved in I thought I would never be able to get used to it. I don't even notice when it comes on anymore.

Ms. Burbridge came to terms with her transition to AL by sheer determination.

I made up my mind when I come here, this was it. I wasn't going to tell my daughters that I'm unhappy if I was. And I just made the best of it, not that I wouldn't rather be in my apartment with help; but I couldn't do it. I couldn't afford it for one thing and [with] this [AL]—they don't have to worry.

Fear

Many people expressed fear of retaliation when they were asked if they had ever communicated their complaints to administrators. Some older adults we interviewed were unwilling to complain, acknowledging the power others hold over their residency there. *"Excessive complaints can only cause people that live in the place trouble,"* were the words of advice given by Dr. Luckingbill, resident of Wetherby Place.

A common complaint among residents willing to assert themselves is how silent everyone else is. Ms. Kates of Wetherby Place made this observation: *"I don't know what's wrong with these people. They complain; I say, 'Well, why don't you [speak up]?'—they're afraid to say something."* Despite her courage, even she acknowledges concerns about jeopardizing her living space. *"I told my daughter, 'They're going to probably throw me out' and I said, 'I don't care, you know. People don't talk.'"*

Silence due to fear of retribution in care or treatment is a very powerful constraint on autonomy, and cannot be underestimated. Residents, and sometimes family members, feel vulnerable in the AL setting. Wendy, whose mother lives at Arcadia Springs, said, "you don't want to complain so much about every little thing because then you feel like it might be taken out on her, you know what I mean."

Although it is frequently noted that in a consumer-oriented setting like AL, "If you don't like it, you can leave," the reality for many residents and their relatives is that another move is not easy or readily undertaken. Suzannah, whose mother lives at Boxwood Gardens, was asked if her mother wanted to move, given all of her complaints. Recognizing just how difficult an undertaking it would be, Suzannah responded, "I think that she [my mother] does not want to move, as much as she complains about the facility, which is daily. And as many things as she does not like there, she has a great fear of trying something else." There are some who have made the move to a different AL setting. But for the most part, financially, logistically, or psychologically, that kind of move is just too difficult for many to undertake, particularly because it is not clear that problems in the current setting would be absent in another AL.

A common fear residents expressed was the fear of being moved to the next level of care, particularly to a nursing home or dementia care unit, a topic we discuss more in depth in Chapter 6. Residents have witnessed triggers for this sort of move, and some will attempt to cover up an incident or change in ability that they perceive places them at risk for such a transition, such as falling or memory loss.

Victoria, the director of Winter Hills, echoes what we heard from many staff members we interviewed:

I have found that people are really good at disguising these changes, sometimes when they first start becoming confused, they know it. I've even had them say to me, you know that's a heck of thing when you're confused and you know you're confused. But they won't be able to finish their sentences, they won't be able to pull words, and they'll say—you know what I mean, you know what I mean? So we're a little more skilled and we key into that, and we'll start looking for other things like putting salt in their coffee instead of sugar.

Staff members are aware of this fear and hiding phenomenon. They are expected to watch for and report these signs of decline, as they have impacts on the AL's staffing, regulatory compliance, and liability issues. These aspects are addressed in more detail in Chapter 6.

Assertiveness

There are many other ways residents assert themselves. Some are quite direct and seem fearless in the way they challenge AL administrators with their concerns or dissatisfactions. Although this aligns with the idea of AL as a consumer-focused care setting, few people expressed their complaints directly. One exceptionally vocal resident we interviewed, Ms. Carson of Boxwood Gardens, kept fastidious, handwritten notes of her grievances, which she would share with the director regularly. These included her disappointment at the lack of assistance in loading her scooter into her car, as we noted earlier in this chapter, as well as concerns about a lack of available medical staff (Chapter 1), adequacy of staff training (Chapter 3), and nutrition (Chapter 4). Our general observation was that, although the complaints were often warranted, Ms. Carson was not endearing herself to the administrators and staff. In the end, she was asked to leave, in part because she resorted to calling the police and fire departments when she felt her concerns were not being adequately addressed by the staff.

As noted in Chapter 2, some residents prominently posted signs on their room doors, a somewhat effective tool used by residents to communicate their wishes to the staff and other residents. At the suggestion of a staff member, Mr. Guarino hung a large black-and-white–lettered "Keep Out" sign on his door in an attempt to keep a wandering resident with dementia, who had been routinely coming into his room at all hours, from entering his room. It worked; she would take one look at the sign and immediately back away. Hank Reichelson, a resident of Greenbriar, compared himself to Rosa Parks, refusing to leave his seat in the dining room when an aide requested him to switch seats: *"I'm not getting up, so go and tell who you want to. I ain't getting up. So they get tough, from this to that. I said, 'Eh.' The next day they said it again. But I didn't care; I wasn't moving."*

Mr. Guarino described the way he would pick and choose his battles. For example, some days when something was not to his liking he said he would *". . . step back and close my eyes. Today's a different story."* He told the researcher, who could see the unmade bed and items strewn about his room where they were meeting to conduct the interview, *"I didn't like the way they were cleaning up here. I would never allow anything like this in my house, and I'm not going to go for it here."*

Other residents chose a more passive-aggressive way to handle their complaints. Ms. Jacobs, as discussed in Chapter 2, objected vehemently to the Greenbriar's new "no food in your room" policy, concerned that the only food available to her in her room were graham crackers served as a snack in the evenings. She warned the staff that eating graham crackers would cause her to have diarrhea.

> *. . . and then you're going to have to have somebody come and clean it up because I'm not going to clean up after a mess that's not my fault. I'm trying to be cooperative, but I can only do what I can do.*

Ms. Jacobs, who is diabetic, decided to pursue a way around the new policy by getting her doctor to overrule the AL's policy. In the meantime, she admitted to sneaking cake and other food items from the dining room to her room to defy the rule.

Others, too, would break rules as a way to deal with these restrictions. Some residents admitted to pretending they were sick, to receive their meals in their rooms and avoid the usual extra fee. Ms. Ames, as mentioned in Chapter 2, said she was willing to abide by the rule to sign out whenever she left, but defied part of the rule by refusing to tell them where she was going.

Frustrated with the performance of the TV cable company with which Greenbriar contracted, Mr. Dugan threatened to withhold his monthly AL payment, until the administrator would agree to change cable companies.

I spoke to the head lady yesterday. I told her I'm not paying my next month's rental because I'm ticked off. And she said, "Well, it's probably a corporate matter." I don't care if it's a corporate matter or not—you shouldn't keep this lousy outfit. They repair something then they screw something else up; so they're not dependable.

A consumer's best recourse, refusal to pay a bill, worked in this case for Mr. Dugan. It got the attention of the administrator.

Advocating

There are some residents who make it a point to speak up for those residents who are more vulnerable. Mr. Guarino, a resident of Arcadia Springs, described an incident where an aide became belligerent with a resident with advanced dementia. After he reported this incident, the aide was fired.

I was down in the living room, and one [of the] staff people got this new guy [new resident]. And she was screaming at him like—his face was here [close] and she's screaming at him. And he's getting worse and worse and worse, and she's screaming louder and louder. You can't do that with these patients—people that live here.... Yeah, [the staff person] strung out her last nerve, but that's too bad. You chose this profession, you know? That's a shame; that [his dementia] is a sickness, you know. He's still a person, that's it—you don't stand there and scream at anybody. She wanted to be on the phone and outside smoking a cigarette.

Mr. Guarino told the supervisor, "*Don't you dare use my name when you're reporting this.*" He was adamant that the AL keep his report anonymous, concerned that there might be some sort of retribution from other staff if he was identified.

Ms. St. John of Boxwood Gardens fought to keep Koko, a well-loved hairdresser, from being replaced, when she heard the new owners were planning to award the contract to a new company.

I went down and said, Koko has been here from the beginning; she knows everybody—and she knows exactly how to do it [hair], exactly the way people wanted. And it's not just putting in a thing [new salon], because a lot of [residents] are handicapped and you've got to be very careful, you know.

Those residents who went out of their way to advocate for a fellow resident were relatively rare. However, more commonly, residents would express in their interviews concern for something they observed. For example, Ms. Pollock who was quoted in Chapter 3, notices the discrepancy in how certain residents are treated. *"I'm afraid everyone doesn't get the same treatment. Just maybe because, well, I might yelp or something, I don't know, you know."* She expressed concern about the physically dependent residents and their well-being, aware of the times the aides have forgotten to bring them down to meals or have left them waiting for long periods of time.

A closer look at these categories of responses to perceived loss of autonomy provides insight into how quality is, in large part, affected by residents' own reactions.

AUTONOMY: THE LITTLE THINGS COUNT

Autonomy, as it is treated in much of the literature, tends to focus on major decisions dealing with finances, health, housing choice, and driving. With few exceptions (Agich, 2003; McColgan, 2005; Roth & Eckert, 2011), the literature fails to note the "everyday" expressions of independence and self-assertion. Although outcomes in major areas certainly matter, many residents in our study already had most big issues settled—a POA had been chosen, the place to live had been decided, and their house and car sold. Residents and staff suggested, instead, that one's sense of autonomy often depends on the little things of daily life. This is in agreement with Agich's assertion that the traditional definition of autonomy for those in long-term care must be reconsidered; it is necessary to acknowledge the significance of things that may seem insignificant to an outside observer (Agich, 2003).

Over the year or more that we knew Dr. Smith, he went from using a hand-powered wheelchair to an electric scooter. This change offered him a freedom he would have never imagined possible after his stroke.

> *It's very easy to use. I'm enchanted with it. It has opened up a whole new world for me just to be able to get out of this place. Four walls, you know, can be very oppressive. I've used it to go—they have this old railroad right of way which runs [between two large cities] and they've turned it into a trail, paved trail. People ride their bikes and hike and jog. And about a mile and a half away, is a beautiful, big drug store, which I have gone to a number of times and gotten snacks and things. As a matter of fact, I went up yesterday, just to go for a ride. And I went down and I got a jar of instant coffee, at a drugstore. Now, isn't that silly?*

Although such a trip might seem trivial to someone in good health and with resources, for Dr. Smith, it is not silly at all. The small things that most people take for granted are anything but small when one's physical ability is challenged. With his electric scooter, Dr. Smith was no longer dependent on the nearby liquor store to bring him cigarettes and a 12-pack of beer, only to have it intercepted at the receptionist's desk. The ability to obtain a cup of coffee in an instant in one's own room is essential to autonomy and self-reliance for Dr. Smith.

Some staff members recognize the importance of what one might refer to as "little things." Roberta, an aide at St. Brigid, made this apt observation.

> The little things—[what] we might think are little things, like cutting their fingernails, or folding up clothes for them, or hanging up clothes for them—it means a lot if you stop to do it for them. Whereas beings you might think just hang up the clothes and go ahead, is no big deal. But to them it is, because maybe they can't do them. Maybe their nails need to be cut and you cut them for them; you know that means a lot to them. Like during the day, if I do little things for them, I know I've done something for them that they want done [and] that they can't do themselves. Whereas, well you just go do it, it means nothing to me and you, but to them it means a lot.

Victoria, the director of Winter Hills, too, understood how these little things make all the difference. She spoke about a recent picnic where they served hot dogs. She is committed to making sure her employees do not dismiss a request, no matter how small.

> These to me, even though they might sound like something little somewhere else, the employees have learned those are big issues to me. A hot dog—what's a hot dog without chopped onions? How can you tell someone we ran out of chopped onions?

TRADING AUTONOMY FOR SAFETY

This chapter demonstrates that, although AL can and sometimes does improve one's independence, many residents identified loss of autonomy as a concern, particularly compared to what they were accustomed to in their former lives. Autonomy, within a context where individuals are dependent on others for help with basic needs, may also be defined differently from when those same individuals had more energy and sharper minds, and were healthier. Loss of autonomy is experienced by residents in varied ways and to varied degrees; asking about it also elicits a variety of responses, some more effective than others.

Many of the common, contested practices of ALs, such as those we have discussed here (limits on coming and going and rationing of sugar, alcohol, and cigarettes) restrict individual freedom and choice. Although it is the expressed intention of AL to foster independence, this value must be balanced with the other key purpose of AL's existence—to provide a safe, healthy, and beneficial environment. Even though the measures, rules, and practices put into place may be restrictive, these are selectively accepted, enforced, obeyed, and welcomed because the people who choose to live in AL expect that they will be looked after should something happen, as is discussed in Chapter 7.

For operators and staff of ALs, many factors contribute to the sometimes restrictive environment. For example, AL is constrained merely by fact of being an institution (see Chapter 2). Managers and owners also live in fear of litigation and under the demands of constantly shifting state regulations, corporate ownership, and financial limitations of running a business, which are all discussed further in the following chapter.

ALs may err on the side of caution, putting into place any number of measures to keep people safe and healthy, thereby constraining their sense of autonomy. But it is within these contexts that many families, residents, and staff come to understand and support the restrictions. We close here by returning to Ms. Powell and her wish for a lock on her door. She comes to a conclusion that demonstrates the imperfect balance between feelings of security and autonomy.

> **Ms. Powell:** *Maybe we'll get locks on the door. But you know what it is, two or three times a night they'll go through here and they'll open your door just to see if you're still in bed or if you're laying on the floor or something. Because you could roll out of bed you know and that.*
>
> **Researcher:** So does that bother you when they come in to check?
>
> **Ms. Powell:** *No, they don't come in; they just open the door and look in.*
>
> **Researcher:** That doesn't bother you, but you'd like a lock on your door.
>
> **Ms. Powell:** *Well, if you put a lock on the door, then they can't look in.*
>
> **Researcher:** So how would you remedy that, what would you do?
>
> **Ms. Powell:** *I don't know. Well, they don't want you to get up and let them know you're okay. In a way it's good and in another way it ain't.*

There are costs, perhaps hidden, to living in AL, and a loss of autonomy is one of those costs. But it may not be as costly as it seems from the outside; as we have learned, many are willing to pay this price for the assistance and peace of mind AL provides.

REFERENCES

Agich, G. J. (2003). *Dependence and Autonomy in Old Age: An Ethical Framework for Long-Term Care.* (2nd rev. ed.). Cambridge: Cambridge University Press.

Dowd, J. J. (1975). Aging as exchange: A preface to theory. *Journal of Gerontology, 30*(4), 585–594.

Funk, L. M. (2010). Prioritizing parental autonomy: Adult children's accounts of feeling responsible and supporting aging parents. *Journal of Aging Studies, 24*(1), 57–64.

Hyer, L. A., & Intrieri, R. C. (2007). Perspective on long-term care: Necessary and unnecessary practices. In L. A. Hyer & R. C. Intrieri (Eds.), *Geropsychological Interventions in Long-Term Care* (pp. 3–36). New York: Springer Publishing.

McColgan, G. (2005). A Place to sit: Resistance strategies used to create privacy and home by people with dementia. *Journal of Contemporary Ethnography, 34*(4), 410–433.

Morgan, L. A., Gruber-Baldini, A. L., & Magaziner, J. (2001). Resident characteristics. In S. Zimmerman, P. D. Sloane, & J. K. Eckert (Eds.), *Assisted living: Needs, practices, and policies in residential care for the elderly.* Baltimore, MD: JHU Press.

Roth, E. G., & Eckert, J. K. (2011). Vernacular landscape of assisted living. *Journal of Aging Studies, 25*(3), 215–224.

Thomas, B., & Blanchard, J. (2009). Moving beyond place: Aging in community. *Generations, 33*(2), 12–17.

Zimmerman, S., Sloane, P. D., Williams, C. S., Reed, P. S., Preisser, J. S., Eckert, J. K.,...Dobbs, D. (2005). Dementia care and quality of life in assisted living and nursing homes [Special issue]. *The Gerontologist, 45*(1), 133–146.

6

External Constraints
Regulations, Rules, and Financial Realities

ORIENTING POINTS

- External factors such as regulations, corporate policy, and funding sources influence the quality balance in assisted living in obvious and subtle ways.
- Regulations provide a baseline for ensuring adequate, safe care but they do not guarantee a high quality of care.

RULES AND REGULATIONS IN AL

In the previous chapter, we addressed the ways autonomy is at times compromised by the assisted living (AL) setting, given its task to care for and protect its residents. In this chapter, we build upon this theme by looking more carefully at the multiple, influential contexts within which the AL must operate. Forces both external and internal to the AL facility influence what takes place within its walls, affecting the quality of everyday life. AL companies or operators are not simply free to offer services in a "free market," an idea consonant with the notion of AL as a consumer-focused sector of long-term care. Instead, rules determined by administrators or owners (whether individual or corporate), and policies imposed by governments, along with the priorities imposed by the costs of providing AL services, constrain what ALs do and how they do it.

Ms. Bachman, a resident of St. Brigid, provides an especially poignant example.

Now last night, I was supposed to have eyedrops in my eyes before I went to bed and nobody was here to do it. But they won't leave the eyedrops in the room for me to do it myself. They said, "We're not allowed to do that." I don't know why I can't, because I've been putting eyedrops in my eyes for a long time and I can do it again. And they tell you, "No, you can't do it." So, then you don't [get the medication]. So I told the day nurse this morning, she says, "Did you have—get an extra pill last night and did you have your eyedrops?" I said, "No." But they don't have anybody—I guess they would have to pay somebody extra [to give the drops]. And they don't want to do that.

Ms. Bachman describes an almost Kafkaesque situation that embodies the tension that results from providers' best intentions to keep her safe, the constraints of regulations against self-administering eyedrops, and bottom line concerns that affect the staff-to-resident ratio. Clearly, St. Brigid's intention is to protect Ms. Bachman from missing a dose or overmedicating herself. Yet, because of the protective measure forbidding self-administering medication, she instead missed receiving in a timely way a medication ordered by her physician. As she suggests, perhaps the shortage of available, qualified staff contributed to her missed eyedrops. We contend here that the array of policies and practices, both through their requirements and through the necessity of managing them, influences quality—but not always in the intended, positive direction.

This chapter addresses how these external constraints are experienced "on the ground." Who or what groups are establishing and interpreting the rules within AL settings? How do those rules play out in provision of care and services day-to-day? What effect do these rules, limits, and regulations have on the quality perceptions of residents, the staff, or others interacting with them? Our goal in this chapter is to shed light onto what may seem like a morass of governmental, in-house, corporate, idiosyncratic, and across-the-board policies, regulations, rules, or unwritten standard practices that exert authority over what happens within the walls of AL. Included in this discussion are the constraints the fiscal bottom line places on AL quality. Money—whether lacking or in abundance—plays a prominent role in how quality is experienced. As we have seen, even those AL settings that are not-for-profit are constrained by budgets.

We begin with the most obvious external constraint within AL, state regulations and the state-government–authorized agencies that have the ultimate power to grant or deny licenses to operate. In this section, we cannot provide a thorough treatment of these regulations; they vary too widely across states, and such a treatment is not compatible with the method or goals of this study. Instead, we focus on the themes related to regulations and oversight that most often came up in the course of our interviews, and therefore those that most impacted the lives of individuals closely linked to daily life within the AL.

STATE REGULATION

Regulations are intended to provide some level of reassurance and confidence in selecting a place of care for people who are vulnerable. For example, Maryland's regulations provide for the authority to deny or rescind an AL's license should "conditions in the facility present an imminent danger to the life, safety, health, or welfare of the residents" (Service agreement requirements, n.d.). Yolanda, a dietary staff member at Arcadia Springs speaks for a number of people when she says she is reassured by the fact that the State has the authority to oversee and take action. Here she compares an in-home care situation with care in a licensed AL setting, where regulatory oversight may limit abuse. "A place like this you have less chance of anything happening, because the State will come in and you can lose your license and you'll never get a job again." Nancy, whose mother lives in Winter Hills, echoes this sentiment, viewing the regulatory powers as a necessary trade-off:

> If there were lots of terrific providers, you wouldn't have to. But unfortunately there are people who make money off of frail individuals and consequently you've got to have regulations that seem prohibitive.

Does Oversight Ensure Quality?

The existence of regulations is no guarantee of high quality care; rather, regulations are meant to provide, at the minimum, protection for vulnerable people from dangerous or poor care. Robert Kane makes the argument that "a regulatory framework provides a floor for quality, but that floor quickly becomes a ceiling" (Kane, 2010).

Yet some of the AL administrators and marketing staff whom we interviewed were quick to cite favorable state inspections as a mark of quality. From their perspective, inspection results were pivotal. This stands in contrast to residents' views, where few mentioned the results of inspections. One of the final questions we posed, very directly, to all of our interviewees was whether they thought the place where they lived, visited, or worked was a quality place. What follows is the answer that Darlene, the administrator of Murray Ridge, gave to this question:

> We try our best, and we've been deficiency free from like the State for years. We haven't had a deficiency. One time the health department, we had a dented can, that's why we didn't get an award. We try real hard. And even when I have a nurse from the pharmacy, she's an RN that comes in and reviews the MARs [Medication Administration Records] and the medicines, she'll tell you. And she would find some mistakes in there, like somebody didn't sign an MAR or something like that. Well, she had said she goes into nursing homes and finds, you know, several mistakes. And you know, she hardly ever finds anything here.

Debra, the director of Wetherby Place, proudly noted how their state surveys improved shortly after she arrived:

> Well, I came in just before the surveyors.... I came in, you know, making sure everything was in place. And the reason I was able to make sure everything was in place [was] because I had just encountered the state survey that had taken place over at [my previous AL]. So survey—they are looking for the same identical thing, so I really didn't have any problems, you know, getting things in place.... I started the CNAs [Certified Nurse Assistants] wearing aprons in the kitchen, you know.... More, being more attentive to the resident, making environmental rounds, going into the rooms, going in and making sure that they have everything they need. So it has been very rewarding because of the quality of care that the residents have received since I've been here.

Debra seemed to be equating positive state surveys with quality. When asked what advice she might give to someone looking to move into an AL, her answer also focused on safety-oriented regulatory issues.

> Well, I would make sure that there is proper staff on 24 hours a day. I would make sure that the food is prepared correctly. I would want to make sure that there is some means of [coordinating], meaning calling if someone fell on the floor—how would you know that they are on the floor? I would be concerned how far away are they [residents] from the nursing station. If there was a fire, how would they get down—you know, elevators? Okay, we have a generator, if the generator goes out what is the means of keeping warm or having hot water? What is the safety of anybody com[ing] in the building? What time at night do they—the doors are locked?

Her perspective, of course, is influenced by her role as the lead enforcer of those regulatory rules and requirements. The state surveys also provide the only tangible measurement that residents and family members can rely on when making choices about where to live; it also provides marketers with a selling point. When we heard residents speak of these things, it was most often because the staff informed them of positive results of a recent state inspection, rather than because meeting these standards mattered to their daily lives.

Perhaps in contrast to Debra's statement, Greenbriar's administrator Jennifer recognized the need to go above and beyond what the State expects and demands in operating an AL setting.

> As the executive director I'm responsible for the overall operations of the community, which consists of financial [oversight], insuring compliance from a regulatory standpoint [and] from a management-human resources standpoint, and insuring that the services we are providing are of a, I would say, a high level of quality of care, the highest level possible that we're able to provide in this type of setting, and, at minimum, meeting the state requirements.

Favorable state surveys and lack of deficiencies may provide some information about a setting, but the picture is incomplete. This is part of an overall argument that this book makes with respect to the complexity and variety of views regarding the key bases of quality.

Down the Nursing Home Path

In contrast to nursing homes, the AL sector is not federally regulated, largely because AL does not receive direct federal reimbursement.[1] AL is, however, regulated at the state level; regulations vary widely from state to state (Assisted Living Workgroup, 2003; Mollica, 2006). Each state, in fact, has its own definition of what kinds of settings constitute AL, as well as differing basic standards of operation and reporting.

The long legacy of nursing home regulation has certainly shaped AL regulations at the state level, with many similar problematic areas addressed in nearly every state. For example, all states require some specific staffing levels, regular health reviews/assessments for residents, contracts between the AL and the consumer (whether the older adult or someone designated by a power of attorney), safety precautions such as building and fire safety (e.g., fire alarms, sprinklers, rules against parking scooters in hallways, and regular drills), and nutritional/food service requirements (e.g., food temperature and balanced, dietician-approved menus).

Ironically, although these elements are described as working to enhance quality, they address only the negative dimension—the avoidance of serious negative outcomes. Meeting state inspection requirements is necessary, but is insufficient to the achievement of quality. Much regulation in AL, as in nursing homes, has been developed in response to incidents or patterns of poor quality and to negotiate the risks inherent in such settings, which serve frail or impaired individuals.

State regulatory bodies have been critical of the AL industry's resistance to the introduction of federal-level regulation. The AL industry views nursing home regulation as unnecessarily adversarial and punitive. They have actively sought to "avoid the mistakes of nursing home regulation" by emphasizing the importance of "outcomes" of care and "customer satisfaction" (Edelman, 2003). Their argument is consistent with the AL principles that promote a more homelike environment and seek to provide residents with choice. AL philosophy essentially

---

[1] Although Medicaid waivers for AL do exist, the federal funds are not given directly to the AL as is the case with nursing homes. Instead, the State runs and operates any Medicaid waiver programs involving AL and is therefore not federally regulated.

advocates a business model where consumers have the power and ability to choose to go elsewhere, should they become unhappy with the current setting. As we discussed in Chapter 5, however, residents tend to be unwilling to directly complain or request changes; they may also feel unable or unwilling to consider a move, given that their next choice may share some of the same challenges. Alice, whose mother lives in Arcadia Springs, was asked if she and her mother had talked about moving.

> No, I mean it would have to get a lot worse for me to do that because, the trauma of moving her—what it would do to her, I mean it would. I mean the people, the CNAs know her. She knows Tara, and you know the kitchen staff knows her and they all treat her good, so I wouldn't. Mom don't know that the sheets weren't changed and she don't get hot because there's no towel in the bathroom, you know. It's me [that does]. And as long as she's calm and happy, you know, I can live with it. And like I said, it could be a lot worse.

Based on the belief that families can "vote with their feet," administrators, such as Darlene at Murray Ridge, think that quality can be measured based on retention. The interviewer asks Darlene, "Do you think this is a quality place?"

> Yeah. I mean, I think that, you know. Like I said, any kind of issues or anything like that are met right away. And I mean, even with the residents' families, they are all happy, because, of course, if they weren't, they would take their families elsewhere.

This response illustrates the way consumer-driven regulation works in theory, but perhaps less so in practice.

Although some have described AL regulation as "nursing home lite," given that the number of requirements and type of enforcement are, thus far, less serious, these regulations do influence daily life and its quality for all participants in AL. Increasingly, AL administrators we interviewed will argue, AL is on the same regulatory path that nursing homes took many years ago, leaving managers and operators to adapt frequently to each newly instituted rule imposed by its state legislature. In many cases, these changes move ALs in the direction of nursing homes.

In her interview, Jennifer Warrenton, Greenbriar's administrator, describes the evolution of AL as it compares to nursing homes and their regulation.

My understanding is that assisted living, when it was developed, it was initially a social model. But over time, as the elderly population continues to grow with the Baby Boomers, and people are living longer and acuity levels [degree of physical or cognitive impairment] are rising, and so it's becoming more of a medical model. At the same time with assisted living, initially it was a social model, my understanding, and perhaps for the more affluent. As people are living longer, funds are running out. So then you have to look at funding. People are asking about [government] funding for staying in the assisted living environment.

Jennifer's comparisons highlight some of the blurry distinctions between nursing home and AL. On one hand, AL's original goal was to provide a less restrictive environment for people with fewer medical needs. But over time, as people age in place, AL has been adapting by increasing its capacity to care for people who in the past would have found themselves in skilled nursing care. Jennifer continues,

I will say when I think about my experience working in nursing homes and working here in an assisted living environment from a quality of care perspective, looking at the individual, the holistic being, I think that assisted living is beneficial from a standpoint. It's not as institutionalized, although we are providing 24-hour care and the acuity level may be a little higher. It's more of a homier environment. We have, I want to say more activities going on and *at this time* the regulations aren't equivalent or as stringent as the regulations in a nursing home environment.

We italicized the caveat Jennifer adds to her observation about current regulations for AL to point out what many people within AL have been saying: AL is soon to become the new nursing home. Joyce Henderson, administrator of Arcadia Springs, expressed concern about the direction things seem to be headed toward:

I'm worried about it, as they slip more and more and more into the State overseeing and pushing more and more medical stuff on us.

And that they're making it more and more nursing home-like. And any day now I think that line is going to get terribly blurred, and it does.

Joyce provides an example and expresses a desire for more flexibility within the regulations, because there are a variety of factors that can sway a decision as to who is admitted or not:

> COMAR [Maryland's state regulatory body], they tell us that we can take Level 3 [highest permitted level of care required] people except for this, that, and the other. But in essence, in reality that person sometimes very well could fit into the AL, but they [the state] won't allow it, because they want that person in a nursing home.
>
> I've walked into some nursing homes—[like] with the last resident that I went out and screened. And I'm looking around at the residents in the nursing home, and I'm going, my God—half of these people could work just as well in my place. Why are they here?

Jennifer from Greenbriar echoes Joyce's concerns that regulatory requirements may be more confusing than they are helpful in determining who qualifies for AL or nursing home care:

> Whereas Maryland...we're a licensed Level 3 community; so when you look at what that means, there is a very fine line between a licensed 3 and a nursing home. In fact, you could have someone that maybe is considered to be a Level 3 and they would be appropriate for a nursing home setting. The Regs [state regulations] here clearly spell out certain areas, such as if someone had a stage 3 [pressure ulcer] or required a vent[ilator] treatment, things of that nature, they should be in a nursing home setting, not in an assisted living setting. But other than that, if you looked at someone who is "total care," if the person could afford to be in this type of setting, then, from a regulatory standpoint, from a productivity labor standpoint, if you can provide them with that service, then they could be in assisted living.

Owners and managers indicated that clarity in regulation and enforcement may be more important than the level of care permitted by the regulations.

Tina Giles, the director of Boxwood Gardens, faces the same difficult determinations as to who should be admitted and who should not. The lack of clarity within the regulations may be seen as an advantage, because of the flexibility it offers. But directors express uneasiness with having to make these critical determinations in an increasingly vigilant but ambiguous regulatory environment. Speaking of the ever-evolving regulatory environment, Tina said,

> It's changing—it's changing—even with the [state option to care
> for very ill individuals] that [AL] has for the residents, where
> I was saying earlier...it allows you that flexibility to bring
> resources in, it also changes to the point to where it's almost
> so identical with...a nursing home. Which makes me wonder,
> what's going to be the difference, you know, after a couple of
> years? It's getting worse—they're getting more stringent on the
> regulations. They're really watching on the state level as to what
> you can and cannot accept. And a lot of things, you look at it and
> it could be a person that's able to walk, talk, move around, do
> just about everything. But depending on what their medications
> [are] and the level and what they're being treated for, it can be
> marked out to where you're not able to have them in a facility.
> And you look at them, and go [say] they definitely don't belong
> in a nursing home, where they don't have a lot of the choices that
> you have in assisted living.

Darlene Hall, director at Murray Ridge, notes these same changes there, with similar concern; however, she characterizes the regulatory changes as allowing for *greater* medical care and aging in place, as opposed to restricting what AL cannot do.

> Yeah, the Regs [state regulations] have changed in the past couple
> years....Like we never could give insulin; we always had to take
> residents who were insulin dependent [and] could do it themselves.
> Now we can give insulin; we can give B12 injections, as long it's
> under [the supervision of] our RN. So yeah, as far as some of
> the regulation changes, the people that we can take [now], we
> couldn't take before. And we can even take some residents [who]
> have ulcers, like bed sores—now [we can accept] a stage 3 [out of
> 4 stages]....We can even really have somebody that is bedridden.
> It's just that we don't want somebody that's bedridden, because

of the fact that of the fire regs, you know; if there is a fire or something—transferring [from bed to wheelchair]—and especially with the girls…that's really a skilled need.…Like they're going to start—they want an RN to be here 7 days a week, or an LPN. They are trying to pass that, so it's continuous changing, where it's going to be like a mini nursing home.

Of particular note here is how Darlene seems to contradict Jennifer, the director of Greenbriar, whose reading of the regulations in terms of accepting people with stage 3 pressure ulcers differed. The actual rule is that, with a proper waiver, the AL can retain a resident who develops a stage 3 pressure ulcer, but AL is not allowed to accept a new resident who has a pressure ulcer of stage 3 or beyond (Level of care waiver, n.d.). The experience directors bring to the reading of the regulations affects the way they interpret the rule. Darlene has only had experience working in an AL environment, whereas Jennifer's nursing home experience perhaps makes her a little more cautious. This divergence in understanding also demonstrates just how difficult some of regulations are to understand and interpret.

The challenge administrators express as they work to meet state regulations may not seem relevant to the quality of life residents experience. However, their decisions to admit or deny certain types of residents affect the social makeup of a place. Or, for example, the accommodations they may be willing (or unwilling) to make for an established resident to remain in AL can determine whether a resident moves on to a nursing home or stays on in his room—a topic we discuss in greater detail later in this chapter.

CORPORATE INFLUENCES

The influence of the administrators, owners, and corporate-office representatives trickles down to each AL, affecting daily life in ways that may not always be recognized by residents. These varied "bosses," as we referred to them in our coding schema, are the people or entities that set the tone and philosophy for the staff, emphasize certain elements of care or services that shape priorities, and determine the composition and character of the staff by their hiring choices.

Administrators in AL chains may have visits from (or to) corporate headquarters, identifying new priorities or policies that broadly apply across disparate settings. Residents were aware when new leadership was hired by "corporate," and knew that this might alter daily routines or priorities (see Chapter 7). Corporate leaders may influence menus, physical elements of the setting, and marketing, or require a certain level of fiscal and quality performance, as evaluated by the state or by "customer satisfaction" surveys. Tina Giles saw both positive and negative aspects to the connection with the corporate.

> I think the positive part that I see with the corporation is that it provides support. I mean there is so much immediate support in the sense that I have the other buildings, the other [directors] there; it's almost like we call each other on a daily basis. You know, I run into this situation, "What have you done? Are you having this problem at your building?" Especially since we share vendors; we use the same food service person, we use the same home health people a lot of the times. Corporate—they have the resources there. There's a corporate representative for the [directors], there's a corporate representative for nursing, there's a senior representative for food services directors....

Her complaint lay in how decisions and policies would be created and applied across all the corporation's settings. The settings under the corporate umbrella varied a great deal—she told us—in size, location, or leadership style, a fact not always recognized by corporate leadership.

> I guess the downfall of the corporation is, well...lot of the things were done up in the corporate office, you know, where [as] reality is down here....some things they do up there...and you may say, OK we're going to try this, this month....[L]et's try this, this month....[W]hen you're just starting it going, they say well, that's not really working, so we're not going to do this....[W]ith each one of our buildings being a little bit different, and sort of having a culture of its own, it may work for [nearby site, but] it may not necessarily work here, and they hear and understand that, pretty much.

Samuel Meadows, director at Wetherby Place, admitted to mixed feelings when asked about how being "under the corporate umbrella" affected his work. For example, Wetherby Place did not participate in the state's Medicaid Waiver program, based on a decision from corporate. Another point of conflict for Samuel was in the strict dietary guidelines dictated by the overarching religiously affiliated corporation. Because the corporation accepted residents of any faith, some of those who did not share the faith complained often, to Samuel, resentful for being denied certain kinds of food as well as alcohol. He, like Tina, expressed gratitude for the support he receives from the corporate and echoes her frustration at some of the confusing "mandates" he receives from them:

> It's good and bad....Monetarily, they have some times where your money all goes up to a big pot, how it trickles down is kind of confusing, to say the least. Because you know you're making money for them and sometimes you know you don't see it....You have corporate assets; you have corporate nurses you can rely on; you have corporate HR you can rely on. [You can have] this kind of parental feel that, if you really get into trouble here with your boots on the ground, you can pick up the phone and get some corporate help. At the same time you always get corporate mandates that you really don't always understand...I kind of have a different perspective than most people. It's kind of schizophrenic. It's good and it's bad.

INTERPRETING, APPLYING, AND ENFORCING THE RULES

Staff Perspectives

It is the director's job to impart policies or rules from corporate, or the owner's job to relay policies to their managers and staff; staff members must then implement these rules "on the ground." Consequently, the staff members responsible for direct care, food service, activities, and other things enact the policies, rules, and "standard practices" throughout their daily routines, which take place more often than not out of the view of supervisory personnel. Circumstances arise where there is no established rule or policy to decide how to deal with a unique situation, such as a fight among family members or residents over the development of a sexual relationship in an individual with dementia. Staff are often put in the position of having to decide what is acceptable and what is not, leaving them to interpret rules/policies/ regulations or create a rule on the fly to address a problem.

With the many nuances involved in deciphering how a regulation plays out in the setting, and considering all the variables, including the traits of the individuals involved, it is no wonder the rules are applied differently, misinterpreted, and/or incorrectly applied from time to time. Jackie, a very seasoned RN from St. Brigid, newly appointed as the AL nurse manager, bemoaned the amount of state regulations for AL. She said it was her greatest challenge when she took on this new role, determining what tasks she must perform versus which duties the licensed practical nurse (LPN) or aides were allowed to perform. She regularly consulted the large book of state regulations on her desk, which held the policies and guidelines to which she must adhere.

Complicating the interpretation of regulations further is the fact that many common practices or in-house rules at times seem to have the force of policy and are frequently mistaken for state or federal regulations. Sister Barbara of St. Brigid tentatively asserted that it was an AL regulation not to allow locks on individual room doors. "I'm not sure on that," she said, second-guessing her assertion, and she then continued, "That's a requirement. I mean, it's not a regulation." Other staff members reported to us, incorrectly, that "the State" makes up all the menus, which is not the case. There are certain dietary and nutritional requirements that must be met, but these food safety and nutritional regulations do not dictate the actual menus.

AL Consumers' Perspectives

Although there were some notable exceptions, many of the residents we interviewed demonstrated a lack of clarity about the rules, often stating things incorrectly or second-guessing rule-related assertions. Anna Ames, for example, said "I noticed that most other places [ALs] did have wheelchair accessible buses, or at least the ones I saw. So I don't know if it's a requirement for assisted living facilities." Lorraine Heilbrun, also of Wetherby Place, referring to differences in single rooms versus double rooms for those living in the Medicaid section, said, *"The law says you're supposed to get equal accommodations."* Dr. Styles said of the Greenbriar, *"I think they have to [do periodic assessments]. Probably state law."* Another resident, Aimee Harris, was under the false impression that participation in exercise and other scheduled activities was a requirement at Boxwood Gardens, where she resided.

Among our interviewees, a number of residents and their family members expressed concern with what they saw as a lack of—or uneven—enforcement of the regulations and rules. Ms. Marshall of Arcadia Springs had been noting recent news stories of neglect and abuse in nearby ALs. This concerned her.

> *There's not enough inspectors, they say. There's not enough people coming around and checking the quarters. If there's a certain number of people [living in the AL], I think they're supposed to. But I know I cut out several editorials that were in the paper about assisted living. I know it's become more of a problem now.*

Enforcement of the rules is often spotty and confusing to residents and family members. The example provided here by Peggy, whose mother lives in Arcadia Springs, demonstrates how these rules are put in place but lack consistency and oversight.

> *Peggy:* They make rules but then they go by the wayside. You know....
>
> *Interviewer:* For example?
>
> *Peggy:* Smoking. Well, the first rule was if you smoked you gave the medicine girl your cigarettes; when you wanted a cigarette you went outside. You were allowed a couple a day. Well, I mean—that didn't last very long. Next thing I know, Mother's got her cigarettes in her bag on her walker....So anyway I talked to [the director] and she mentioned the lighter and I said, you know what, that never entered my head. I mean even dummy me, didn't think of it. That's what she shouldn't have....She's supposed to hand it back. Well, how long did that last? Two weeks. I'd go in there and she'd have cigarettes in her bag and/or a lighter and go out.

Both Ms. Rohan, a resident of Wetherby Place, and her daughter Laurel expressed a great deal of concern for what they described as a lack of accountability and action on the part of Wetherby Place and its staff. *"I would first, make rules,"* Ms. Rohan said, when asked what she would do differently if she were in charge. *"And make sure that everybody follows those rules."* She continued, *"I'd make rules for the patients as well as the help. And make it a strict, disciplined, place. I think that would improve it."* Ms. Rohan went on to describe a troubling event she witnessed. Ms. Rohan was among several residents who noticed another woman calling for help, pulling on her call button. All the while this was happening, an unpopular LPN did not answer the call button. Laurel describes the LPN as "loud, talks in a booming voice, in a berating way. But she stood in this lobby and laughed and mocked this woman [who was calling for help], and it was upsetting to everybody that knew what was going on." Ms. Rohan interjected,

> *And she [the resident] had a stroke right out there—her brain went. She said, "They're killing me. They're killing me." And the [staff members] didn't realize what was happening and they laughed—this one nurse. All the rest of us were sitting around observing.*

Laurel continued, "[The residents who witnessed this were] mortified."

The lack of confidence and lost sense of security Ms. Rohan and her daughter expressed as a result of this incident led them to conclude that more must be done to protect residents. Laurel feels unable to speak out for fear her mother may be harmed in retaliation. Staff members who should be fired—she said—are instead "written up" and are quickly back on the job. According to Laurel,

> Everyone has accidents, every person, we're human. But when the staff doesn't have the integrity to apologize or own up to incidents—where they make a mistake and then you say something. In [Wetherby Place] they're counseled—something is put in their [staff member's] file and then they come back and they punish [the residents]. It's like hazing the residents for saying something.

Laurel's concerns echo what we heard from residents and other family members, as discussed in Chapter 5. Laurel strategized, "I pick and choose my battles. If I contact a person, it's in a positive regard. I really don't feel like I want to make my mother a target." Laurel suggested the need for a "Bill of Patients Rights" to protect people who are senile. But from what she and her mother have observed, even improper and perhaps fireable offenses did not lead to any meaningful action by the AL's management.

Enforcement, implementation, and interpretation can vary a great deal among AL settings. Mr. Guarino of Arcadia Springs, in addition to telling the story in Chapter 5 about the verbally abusive staff member, relates another incident where he watched as a medication aide left the medication cart unattended and opened one evening in a public space. He watched as a resident with significant cognitive impairment approached the unattended cart, helped herself to the little snacks on the cart, and returned to her card game. He tried unsuccessfully to stop the woman from going to the cart. Fortunately, she did not help herself to any of the little cups of medications or the blister packs of pills stacked in the drawers of the open cart. *"I told that story the next day and that's it; I haven't seen that particular nurse here since."*

The managers, executive directors, and others who hire and fire have a big influence on the character and effectiveness of the staff. Tara, for example, compared her fellow aides at Arcadia Springs with her coworkers from her prior job at a nursing home. The nursing home aides, especially those of the day shift, she described as, "real rude and not as nice as they are here." There, she said, "it seemed like they'd hire almost anyone, and they just didn't care, because they [aides] wanted a paycheck, and that was it. Like here, I think everybody is almost all well educated and have a good head on their shoulders," she said of her coworkers at Arcadia Springs.

Moving to the Next Level

As discussed previously, administrators play a major role in interpreting regulations regarding when a resident may stay or when they must leave. Although Maryland has three levels of care within its state regulations, there is a lot of leeway in the way the assessments placing individuals into these levels are conducted and interpreted. The movement from one level of care to the next, or from one unit in the AL to another (e.g., to a specialized dementia care unit) is often fraught with disagreement and distress. Each setting has its own set of "triggers" or requirements that will indicate when a resident needs to move. Even with these sorts of house rules, exceptions abound. Those in charge at the facility level, as well as at the corporate level, informed by a set of state regulations and guidelines, determine what they can or cannot manage in terms of adequately and safely staffing for higher medical needs.

There was a lot of variance among settings in our study as to what would trigger a move. For example, in the case of St. Brigid, an AL licensed for Level 1 care only, the triggers that indicated an imminent move to one of the adjacent nursing units were the need for help with bathing and managing medications and the inability to do one's own laundry. Other settings such as Winter Hills "welcomes Level 3 care, including residents with catheters and other high-level needs, and can manage to keep residents as they become more frail," according to an informal conversation with Victoria, Winter Hills's director.

> Victoria did note, however, that the ability of a resident to stay at Winter Hills has a lot to do with the capability of the staff. She gave the example of a hypothetical "large man," who would have to leave if the staff could no longer pick him up [should he fall or not be able to rise from his bed or chair]. She contrasted this with a small woman who might have a very high need for assistance in many areas, but who would be able to stay in Winter Hills if the staff were able to manage her and continue picking her up.

At St. Brigid, many of the residents believe that when their medications are "taken away" from them, it is the first step toward being required to move to one of the nursing units. In an interview with Jackie, a nurse administrator at St. Brigid, she said she spends a great deal of time trying to assuage residents' fears about moving to a higher level. *"Do I have to go now?"* they ask when the staff members require them to turn in their medications to be centrally managed. But, despite her words of assurance, residents are keenly aware of signs that precipitate a move to the next higher level, moves that are enforced by the nuns. Jackie explains the policy at St. Brigid.

> I, around every three months, evaluate whether a resident is able to take their medicines or not. And spend time with them if we have to take the medicines away, because of maybe cognitively they're

not as good as they were, or they can't see it correctly, or they don't know why they're taking it. And we just explain to them, because they're afraid that that might push them one more step to the nursing unit. So we explain that it's for their good, for their safety.

Because the St. Brigid AL unit provides only Level 1 care, there is a steady stream of movement to higher levels within that campus. These transitions frequently become sources of conflict between residents and those who enforce the moves; in the end, residents almost always agree to the move.

After a field visit to St. Brigid, a researcher recorded her notes from an encounter with a resident who had recently been moved to the next level:

> A former AL resident from [the next level up], a more advanced nursing unit within St. Brigid, was wheeling a fellow resident in to see her old room in the AL. The room is directly across from Ms. Harding's and it was empty except for a bed and a night stand. The resident said she was forced to leave by Sister Barbara—she expressed genuine dislike for her, but followed that by saying, "God bless her anyway." I asked her why she was forced to leave, and she said Sister Barbara kept accusing her of wearing soiled clothing and felt that because she wasn't doing her own laundry (she paid someone else to do it), she wasn't able to keep her clothes clean. So she was forced to leave against her will.

This exchange between the researcher and former AL resident was overheard by Ms. Harding, who later told the researcher that "*this resident had been falling fairly often—not over rugs or objects—just falling. And so they were concerned about her health and that is the real reason she was moved.*" In short, some of the criteria that residents believed to place them at risk for moving didn't necessarily match with those used by staff and administrators to make these decisions. Nonetheless, residents are watchful as they note which—and when—fellow residents move on to the next level and the apparent reasons for this move. As we discussed in Chapter 5, for some residents this is a cause for anxiety and prompts them to hide certain needs as a way to avoid a move.

When residents decline physically and/or cognitively, the care aides also have a big influence on how long residents can remain. For example, some aides report having to do extra work for certain residents; in some cases they are willing to overlook this burden, because that person is especially liked by the staff. Often, the complaint we heard came from direct care staff; administrators are willing to retain people with significant impairments, beyond what the aides feel is in their capacity to manage. These aides are aware of the economic pressures shaping the administrator's decisions; as one aide noted: "If anybody they want to come in, they say, 'Hey, as long as you have the money.'" Some aides expressed concern for their professional credentials or their job security, should such a resident be injured on their watch. They felt insufficiently trained to meet the higher level of severity of illness shown in the residents that their ALs were admitting and retaining.

The Health Insurance Portability and Accountability Act

The Health Insurance Portability and Accountability Act (HIPAA; U.S. Department of Health and Human Services, n.d.) is a federal law devised to address several goals, among them to protect each individual's health information privacy. HIPAA is invoked with great frequency by both staff and residents, though with differing attitudes. The AL staff are carefully instructed to keep personal health information confidential. Some adhere to this more strictly than others, but the law is well known among most aides and among all the licensed nursing staff. What this means to the people who reside in AL is that they are often kept in the dark about the whereabouts and status of the people with whom they share daily life in the collective AL environment. Officially, residents cannot be told whether or why a neighbor or friend is in the hospital, unless the neighbor supplies a written waiver.

Perhaps the most cited consequence of HIPAA was the way deaths and hospitalizations were not communicated or were poorly communicated within the AL. Some ALs will place a single rose in the lobby, perhaps with a photo of the recently deceased resident. This will be the only "announcement" that the death occurred. In an interview with a resident's daughter, she said she finds it "interesting" how residents' passing is not announced:

> Mom says they just sort of disappear and they don't really tell you when someone dies.... She'll say, well, her good friend that was at

the table…went off to a nursing home or into the hospital and she's in bad shape. I said, "Well, do you think she's still living?" She says, "I don't know. And believe me, it won't be announced."

Many people are not aware of the federal law that is behind this lack of open communication. One resident thought maybe the AL wants to avoid getting the "*bad reputation*" they would have if they were to make it known that residents were leaving for the hospital or dying. Another resident surmised that the reason staff would not share information was to protect residents from any emotional distress:

Because one day they are sitting at the table next to you and the next day they are not there, and you just have to guess and it gets around by word of mouth. But at first they didn't announce it. I guess they thought it would upset people.

Michelle, the director of marketing at Boxwood Gardens, could understand residents' curiosity and concern. "…They are concerned it's one of their friends," she said. When asked if she shares any information with residents, she responded:

No, because of HIPAA, and this is how I try to explain it to them [the residents] and obviously we can't stop them from seeing who is wheeled out on a stretcher. If they rush down to the lobby and they see someone going out, I say to them, "You and your family probably wouldn't want everyone to know your business if you had to go to the hospital. I don't know anything; hopefully she'll be home soon."…I wouldn't tell someone else—because it's kind of gossipy.

From the perspective of a resident, this kind of secrecy about the people they live with day-to-day, and sit with at every meal, can be upsetting and contradict a philosophy within AL that this place is home and the people who live there are "*like family.*" If so, some residents have asked, why then should they be kept in the dark about their friends' well-being? Ms. Carson, a resident at Boxwood Gardens, is aware of the HIPAA law and accepts its clear restrictions.

It's not allowed for us to know if someone is ill here—what happened to them all of a sudden when they don't show up any more. We're not really allowed to know what happened to that person. Somebody else might know because one of the children came in and told them, or something like that. But officially we can't ask any questions about the health or the whereabouts of any other resident.

A good example for how confidentiality is handled in a way that gives residents the possibility of controlling their HIPAA-restricted personal information comes from one facility: that AL gives every resident the opportunity to sign a waiver to allow the staff to communicate with fellow residents about the signee's health status, should it change suddenly.

THE FINANCIAL CONTEXT

Financial constraints have a significant influence on quality in AL. Its effect is felt at nearly every turn, from fear of litigation to the need to keep beds filled. Decisions about policy, practice, and day-to-day rules are influenced by the monthly budgets of the facilities themselves and by the budgets of the residents who pay to live there. The amount of money available to an individual (resident or family member) or the setting's budget can limit or expand options and range of service. Staff are also affected by the amount of pay and benefits a setting provides, which directly influences staff turnover, retention, and quality of workers.

Family members become particularly savvy as they work through policy-based financial supports such as Medicaid and Veterans Administration (VA) benefits. Kathy, whose father lives in Greenbriar, applied for the VA's "Aid and Assistance." Once it was granted, he could afford to move out of his shared room into a private studio. What benefits one qualifies for is an issue for families and residents. "You know that you can call the VA and 80% of the people [at the VA] don't know about the program." Kathy said in her interview, demonstrating how difficult it is to get information. In her father's case, because the extra monthly income afforded him a private room, her father, she said, was much happier.

Prior to moving in, most AL marketing staff will discuss the issue of money with the prospective resident and/or family members. Samuel

Meadows, Wetherby Place's director, recommends sitting down with a calculator and "try to figure...out how much time are you going to have in that assisted living." This is absolutely necessary, he said, "if it's not a subsidized facility and it's a private paid facility, like most of them are."

Medicaid and AL is a subject of much debate. Each individual state determines how it will allocate and manage federal Medicaid benefits. In Maryland, AL was provided a certain number of slots, with the vast majority of Medicaid recipients going to nursing homes. Because AL has been primarily private pay, the ALs that accept Medicaid as payment are few and far between. In this study, three had some shared rooms available for Medicaid-qualified residents. However, during the time of the study, Arcadia Springs cut its number of Medicaid spots from 12 to 7 because of a new rule that lowered their reimbursement; some Medicaid residents were compelled by Medicaid to spend their daytime hours in a nearby senior center. Joyce, the administrator at Arcadia Springs, noted that her costs did not change simply because a resident was not in the building during some of the daytime hours, yet her reimbursement for those residents had been cut.

Although it is possible to find an AL that will accept Medicaid, getting the waiver from the State to use Medicaid reimbursement for AL is a challenge. Given this reality, Michelle, a marketing director at Boxwood Gardens, said her focus needs to be on identifying individuals able to afford her AL's services, including Medicaid. When asked if Boxwood Gardens accepts Medicaid, Michelle answers, "We do, we take the Medicaid Waiver, but right now in Maryland it's about a two-year wait list....I just called the waiver service and there are 7,500 people on that list right now."

Fortunately for Peggy, Ms. Hill's daughter, she was able to get her mother's Medicaid approved for a move from the nursing home to Arcadia Springs, though it took many months of working through paperwork, caseworkers, and social workers. "It was a terrible thing. I mean, you know, nobody knows what they're doing. I'm telling you nobody knows what they're doing." Now living in a shared room in Arcadia Springs, Peggy's mother must be reapproved for Medicaid every year. Reapproval based on financial need is never a problem, she said; it's the medical approval that is more likely to be an issue. Peggy's mother was denied the year after she moved into Arcadia

Springs; Medicaid determined Ms. Hill's stay in AL to be "medically unnecessary." With the help of a psychiatric evaluation and hearing in front of a judge, this decision was eventually overturned. But it is this uncertainty that keeps Peggy from exploring alternative options for her mother. Both Peggy and her mother have complaints about the care she is receiving at Arcadia Springs. Peggy says,

> I might investigate some, [but] I'm just scared to death of the medical assistance stuff [losing her Medicaid benefit]. I mean I know I would not have any assistance from my brothers if we would have to go to private pay. That means out of my pocket. I'm going to have to pay what—$4,000 a month plus all her little expenses. There is no way. So I have to stay with a facility that is going to give her the medical assistance.

Because the Medicaid waiver waiting list is so long, most people never make it off that list. Some ALs, especially those that suffer from low census, have been willing to "work" with established residents and their families to make the finances work. The resident may be offered a shared room at a lower rate, for example. One setting from a previous study we did would accept the Medicaid reimbursement rate from a resident who had spent down his assets as a way to keep him there, though it meant moving the person to a shared room. These efforts are all made to prevent a move to a nursing home, where care would be virtually guaranteed coverage by Medicaid. For those ALs that are not census challenged or are profit-driven, there may be few options for the person who has spent down her money. Residents are often forced to leave.

Dee Carsin, whose aunt lived in Murray Ridge, was faced with this difficult situation. Once her aunt's money ran out, Darlene, the administrator, suggested they get her aunt on the Medicaid waiver list. "She was like number 4,000 and something," Dee said. "I mean, she was nowhere near the top of the list."

> …So we kind of came up with a plan. Darlene suggested that if you can get her into a nursing home for like 30 to 45 days and then have her come back, it bumped her up to the top of the list.… You know, so when we told her she was going, she got hysterical. She started crying, you know and said please don't make me go, I don't

want to die among strangers. So my husband and I felt, alright, we'll pay it.

Her aunt eventually moved up the list to number 1,500 but there was no guarantee she would live to receive the benefit. Dee said:

> I hope she lives another three years just to get some money out of them. [laughter] I mean, you know, for God's sake she's going to be 100 years old! What do you have to do? [laughs] And I've written to everybody. I have just, you know, and there's just no way to do it.

Dee chose not to force her aunt to make the short-term nursing home stay in order to jump the list. "We have to sleep at night," she said of her and her husband's decision to pay for their aunt's monthly stay at Murray Ridge.

> The State just doesn't fund [Medicaid for AL] sufficiently. They throw a little money at it and that opens up some slots. But basically you have to wait for somebody to die to get [them] off the list so your name goes up higher.

WHEN REGULATIONS AND RULES CAUSE HARM

A surprising outcome of this study is that ALs may sometimes compromise resident quality by their very efforts to promote a safe and more homelike setting. For example, many ALs require all residents to give over their medications to be kept and distributed by trained staff. The opening story of this chapter, featuring Ms. Bachman's eyedrops, is a good example of how a rule could, in fact, cause harm. Ms. Carson, a resident of Boxwood Gardens, explained how useful it was for her to have access to her pill bottles.

> *When I used to have my pills at my bedside when I was home, I knew what they looked like and I saw the label. But [here] they take them away from us and bring them down in the cup, and we have to try to go over them, if they have the time. And then the pharmaceutical companies change the shape or the color, and then you have to ask, "Well, what are the milligrams? What is this pill for?" It's very confusing, and they [staff dispensing medications] don't know half the time themselves.*

Having the staff keep medications to manage, refill, and administer is assumed to be the safest way to control for overdosing, incorrect dosing, or missing a dosage. A one-size-fits-all rule also reflects the relatively high rates of dementia in AL. Having everyone's medications managed by the AL avoids problems when cognition prevents success at self-managing and doesn't stigmatize those unable to handle their own medications effectively. Even if a resident is capable of managing her own medications, unlocked doors might permit a confused wanderer access to those medications. Certainly, some residents would appreciate and could benefit from being brought into the process of managing medications more directly or given more control over their medications.

Another example of how a safety measure or precaution is counterproductive is from Ms. Isaacs, a woman who, after a fall and stay in the hospital, was specifically ordered by the staff not to leave her room by herself. They recommended she stick to her wheelchair at all times, but despite this order, she began to walk on her own.

> *Ms. Isaacs:* Well, I started walking with my walker. I have to get out of this chair. . . . I can't sit in this chair for 24 hours a day. But anyway, I started walking the halls. First day I could walk just to where the three chairs are out there [hallway], and sit down and come back to my room. And each day I started walking more and then started circling around, around and around. And then one morning, they always take me to my meals in the wheelchair. So one morning I thought, you know, I'm going to go get my breakfast. I'm going to walk down, because I knew my way around by that time. So I got my breakfast. They had told me not to ever go out by myself. Well, I did anyway. And I got along fine, and I've been walking to my meals ever since.
>
> *Interviewer:* Really? Were they surprised?
>
> *Ms. Isaacs:* Nobody ever said anything, I don't think [laughs]! Well, they're busy with other things. If you don't make a big to do about it, they don't really know what you're doing.

Another example of how a safety measure impedes autonomy is the carpeted floors found in most ALs. Dr. Smith complained about the drag on his wheelchair from the carpets.

I get enough exercise running this wheelchair up and down these damn rugs, if I may use that expression. It's like trying to pedal across glue, you know. Well, hospitals have tile floors because they have to wheel these gurneys and things back and forth. And I could really stand to have tile floors around here. And you know that café area is a hardwood floor. I zoom across that, like somebody put a rocket in my pants or something. I zoom and then I hit the rug. . . . Well, I think they're afraid of people taking spills, falling.

The original intent of AL was to look as little like a hospital or nursing home as possible. Carpeting is less institutional-feeling and creates a softer landing in case of falls. But in terms of mobility, the ease with which it allows someone to wheel his own chair, uncarpeted floors might be a more practical choice. In the early years of AL, there were not nearly as many wheelchairs or walkers as there are today.

Common practices in AL, such as the examples described earlier— restricting mobility, mandatory management of medications, and carpeting—have developed over the years in the name of safety, even as AL has sought to provide more freedom, independence, and a home-like setting.

QUALITY BALANCE—NEGOTIATING THE RULE OF AUTHORITIES WITH RESIDENT QUALITY

Given the power of these externally driven forces, how then does the AL, a resident, or family member find a happy balance? The answer, broadly speaking, may be in AL's ability to remain as flexible as possible. Flexibility is built into the way AL is regulated, by design. Although ALs across the states typically use a set of parameters for admission and retention, they do "allow individual residences to determine whom they will serve and what services will be provided within the parameters set by regulation." The state agencies responsible for licensing AL and other residential options have adopted regulations that allow a broader level of services to meet the needs of residents as they age in place (Mollica, 2005). An administrator from an earlier study articulated how she viewed her role as a decision maker.

> …things are not clear-cut—I mean every case is different—every resident is different, every staff member, every situation is just so different. And you just have to make so many judgment calls and decisions and it's not like, black and white. So they try to help you with that by giving you lots of tools and resources and things to make things clear for you. But when it comes down to it—it's just—taking every case individually.

She recognizes how not having universal rules may cause some confusion and uncertainty, but understands that it is also what makes it possible to treat each person as an individual.

We discovered examples of how some ALs are able to balance rules and regulations with resident quality in such a way as to promote true options and control over important decisions. Some settings will draw up informal agreements, sometimes referred to as negotiated risk agreements (Wilson, Burgess, & Hernandez, 2001). Although these agreements may not be contractual or binding in the legal sense (Carlson, 2003), they give the resident and family members the ability, for example, to opt out of the nightly checks, or they can allow a resident to leave the building freely. Often, risk agreements are entered into when an AL is uncomfortable with a resident's behavior or level of need and may have otherwise been asked to leave. In this interview excerpt, Nancy, whose mother is a resident at Winter Hills, explained how she handled a similar situation.

> I finally said to [the director], what do I need to, in essence, absolve you of in order for her to stay there. And part of it was my mother was having problems with her legs. She wasn't sleeping at night. She was doing a lot of wandering in the building. They were concerned of an elopement risk, or her wandering outside. I was not, so I said OK, what if I write something that says if my mother should leave the building and break a hip or whatever, or bottom line is she's walking around, if she leaves the building, I know that's a possibility and I'm willing to take the risk for that.

Many residents, family members, and staff shared in common a general uncertainty about the rules and regulations. This is not surprising, given the complexity of the many factors involved and the AL industry's resistance to black and white, universal standards. Whereas everyone agrees that the goal is quality of life for older adults who reside in AL, staff rules, state regulations, and finances and financial programs cannot adequately ensure quality.

The external constraints laid out in this chapter necessarily impact quality. In the next chapter, we look more closely at the ways people react and adapt within this context and explore the challenges to quality when so much within an AL is subject to change. Becky, whose mother lives in Winter Hills, aptly summarizes the challenge to providing a quality AL experience, given all the competing demands. When asked, "If you were in charge; if you were the director, [what would you do differently?]," her response was definitive:

> Oh, my! I wouldn't want to be the director. I'm sure that the head of it, you've got paper work like crazy, the health department, you know. I can't—how can, you have to be efficient, and you've got to make money. It is still a business and yet you've got to care about the residents.

REFERENCES

Assisted Living Workgroup. (2003). Assuring quality in assisted living: Guidelines for federal and state policy, state regulation, and operations. Retrieved October 5, 2010, from http://www.theceal.org/ALW-report.php

Carlson, E. (2003, Spring). In the sheep's clothing of resident rights: Behind the rhetoric of "negotiated risk" in assisted living. *NAELA Quarterly.*

Edelman, T. S. (2003, Spring). Enforcement in the assisted living industry: Dispelling the industry's myths. *NAELA Quarterly.*

Kane, R. T. (2010). Reimagining nursing homes: The art of the possible. *Journal of Aging & Social Policy, 22*(4), 321–333.

Level of care waiver. (n.d.). Code of Maryland Regulations. Retrieved January 27, 2011, from http://www.dsd.state.md.us/comar/comarhtml/10/10.07.14.22.htm

Mollica, R. L. (2005). *Aging in place in assisted living: State regulations and practice.* Washington, DC: American Seniors Housing Association.

Mollica, R. L. (2006). *Residential care and assisted living: State oversight practices and state information available to consumers* (AHRQ Publication No.

06-M051-EF). Rockville, MD: Agency for Healthcare Research and Quality.

Service agreement requirements. (n.d.). Code of Maryland Regulations. Retrieved January 20, 2011, from http://www.dsd.state.md.us/comar/comarhtml/32/32.03.03.10.htm

U.S. Department of Health and Human Services. (n.d.). Health information privacy. Retrieved September 16, 2010, from http://www.hhs.gov/ocr/privacy

Wilson, K. B., Burgess, K. L., & Hernandez, M. (2001). Negotiated risk agreements: Opportunity or exploitation? *Ethics, Law, and Aging Review, 7,* 59–79.

7
Broadening Our Perspectives on Quality
Change Over Time in the Quality Balance

ORIENTING POINTS

- Quality is a moving target, because both residents and assisted living settings change over time.
- Changes in assisted living settings at many levels influence the quality of daily experience for residents.
- The resident's initial quality balance or imbalance changes as the resident, the setting, or both, change over time.

QUALITY AS A MOVING TARGET

We interviewed David Levenson, a retired senior executive of a publishing firm, in June, 2006 at Wetherby Place. A double amputee, his health had improved since he arrived there, moving from Level 3 (highest care needed) down to Level 1. Most important to him was regaining his capacity to manage bodily care tasks, which reduced his embarrassment and sense of dependence. In his untaped interview shortly before his 80th birthday, he was emphatic about recovering his health, his ability to walk with his prostheses, and, ideally, finding a female companion to enable him to return to life in a seniors apartment complex. Mr. Levenson didn't believe he belonged in assisted living—he enjoyed challenging himself intellectually as well as physically. An interview with Fred Braskey showed his respect and admiration for Mr. Levenson; and Dr. Luckinbill, another of the small group of men at Wetherby Place, said, "*[H]e's a very smart guy, probably smarter than I am.*" Mr. Levenson also was popular with the ladies. According to Ms. Rosenstein, another Wetherby Place resident, he had a lady friend at Wetherby Place, and he also flirted with her about the sexiness of her long, blonde ponytail. Ms. Rosenstein, interviewed six days after Mr. Levenson, told us that he was then in the hospital. Mr. Levenson developed sepsis associated with one amputation site, which aggressively spread and killed him within two weeks. His passing was noted by others, who missed his forceful presence among the residents.

Although most of the attention to change over time in assisted living (AL) has focused on residents' health changes, particularly declines in physical or cognitive functioning (often unfolding at a much slower pace than in the story described earlier), our research shows that (1) resident changes are more varied than just declining health and, importantly, (2) AL settings themselves are subject to significant changes that influence the quality of experiences of residents over time. Although ALs appear stable when seen daily in the community or visited prior to selecting a setting for oneself or a relative, over the course of a year or even several months many AL settings experience subtle and major changes. These changes may reshape the AL's service offerings, alter the social environment created collectively by the residents, modify the leadership style, and result in reactions to a shifting external environment. Because our research involved interviewing staff and residents living and working in AL settings over approximately 18 months, it was possible to observe changes in the AL settings themselves and their external environments, including competitors and regulators. Some ALs are surprisingly stable, but others encountered small, cumulative changes or faced major ones, resulting in changes in the quality of residents' daily lives. The focus in this chapter is on change over time in AL and the ways in which the quality balance for residents, ideally present when a new resident moves in, can erode over time through varied changes in the residents themselves as well as in the AL setting.

Each quality evaluation in AL, whether conducted by the owners of a freestanding or chain of ALs, by a researcher, or, informally, by a resident or visiting family member, is a snapshot view of quality at a single moment in time. Although these assessments are useful, our research (with a somewhat longer view that included work in our study sites and in nine other AL settings since 2001) reveals that the dynamics of ALs over time contribute substantially to how well a resident's needs and wants are met within a particular setting (Eckert, Carder, Morgan, Frankowski, & Roth, 2009). In short, the resident's quality balance may shift not simply because that resident changes, but also because the AL setting itself is evolving through time in ways that influence that balance.

CHANGES WITHIN RESIDENTS

Decline in a resident's health—more specifically, the resulting growth in the need for personal care, medical services, monitoring, and mobility assistance—is a familiar topic in discussions of AL, because it increases the odds of residents moving to a higher level of care (Eckert et al., 2009; Wolinsky, Callahan, Fitzgerald, & Johnson, 1993). Our interviews identified residents who were challenged by health and cognition changes, many of which could eventually lead to a move from AL to a dementia care setting or a nursing home.

Mr. Leland exemplified those residents who noticed changes in themselves and attempted to cope with them, rather than hiding them.

I have more trouble with names now than I ever did. I only ask for the first name. I don't want to complicate things. . . . I can remember most of them. I jog my memory like while I'm eating in there [dining room]—I'll say, there's Joe, there's Mary, there's—you know, and go through . . .

Whereas Mr. Leland did not require extensive help due to his memory problems when we interviewed him at St. Brigid's, some residents, such as Mr. Levenson, discussed in the opening story, experienced more sudden or more severe changes that altered their daily lives in AL or resulted in their moving to a facility with a higher level of care. Some changes were gradual progressions, whereas others were punctuated with acute incidents, like falls or illnesses, which sometimes required hospitalization.

Unexpected Changes

Declining health seems to be expected, but less-expected changes also arose among residents we interviewed. One type involves an improvement in health, as was the case with Carol and Bob Moyers. These married professionals, younger than average AL residents, were recovering from brain injuries after an auto accident. During their time in AL they were exercising vigorously, hoping to regain their prior autonomy, dismiss their respective Powers of Attorney, and return to a more normal life outside AL. Anna Ames also was improving. Although not planning to leave her unit in the Greenbriar, she described her recovery of physical function following a major spinal cord injury several years earlier. After hospitalization, rehabilitation, and a prior stay in AL, she had moved in with her daughter for a while.

> *And I stayed with my daughter from 6 to 8 months, I think. Yeah, about 8 months, and then I came here. Because, you know progressively I just got better and better, and I really wanted a place of my own. And, as far as everybody was concerned, this is as close as I can get to my own place again, but close to my children.*

Later she added,

> *I like Greenbriar—[it] helps me feel like I'm getting more like what I was. I'm becoming more like myself. And it gives me a little bit more freedom than even when I was with my daughter. Because, even though she had the same kind of basic set up, and she had somebody cooking for me and all that stuff....like I said, [being here] it's the security and safety and peace of mind for her.*

Following the move, neither mother nor daughter had concerns that Ms. Ames's needs for daily assistance might be unmet by irresponsible home care aides when the daughter needed to travel on business. Other unexpected changes, including those relating to adaptations to the new setting and shifting attitudes, are discussed later in this chapter.

Changing Attitudes and Perceptions

Several residents we interviewed emphasized changing their own attitudes or perceptions over time as key to a quality experience in

AL. In Chapter 6 we discussed how attitudes and acceptance can be employed to deal with reduced autonomy. But changes in perceptions of oneself or one's situation also are part of the dynamic of change in individuals that shifts the quality balance. Moving to AL, as well as changes that occur afterward, often forced older adults living there to face their own aging, and the challenges that come with it. Fran Spivey, for example, who'd had an active social life in her prior apartment, indicated that her view of life at Arcadia Springs was influenced by her sense of self. *"I'm old, there's no doubt about that, but I mean . . . I don't know how to act old. I'm used to being around crowds. But it seems like [where I lived before] people were more alive or something."* Mr. Cohen said of Wetherby Place,

> *. . . I'm still here and I don't see any prospects of leaving here. It's just one of those things, when you get to a certain age you just have to put up with assisted living, which is what we get here. So that's where I am and that's why I'm here and that's how the prospects look to me for getting out of here.*

Typical among the more enthusiastic was Barbara Hayduk, who described Murray Ridge in mostly positive terms during her interview, despite some reservations. She decided to make the best of a situation that was not her choice or preference. When asked to elaborate on what she liked about the place, she said,

> *Ms. Hayduk: Well, it's homey, you know. People are friendly. They keep it nice and clean. The food is pretty good, which is unusual for a place where you have to stay that you're not used to. Everybody treats us good—I don't have any complaints at all really. I don't know if anybody else does, but we seem to get along with everybody. . . . Everything seems to be all right. Of course I miss being home, but what are you going to do—there comes a time in life when you've got to make a change—you've got to do it.*
>
> Researcher: If somebody—if one of your friends was thinking about moving into an assisted living, what advice would you give them? Things to look for, things to stay away from. . . . ?
>
> *Ms. Hayduk: Well, nothing really—I mean just go along with whatever's there, and make the best of it. Everybody treats you OK—there's no reason why you can't make it. It's up to you, your attitude.*

Sometimes surprising changes became part of adapting to AL, such as those reflected by Fred Braskey, who indicated that his attitudes on race had shifted considerably since moving to Wetherby Place. Although he was required to work with people of other races during his career, his prejudices hadn't shifted until he lived in AL, where most direct care staff were immigrants.

> *Mr. Braskey: I said at one time I wouldn't work with blacks. But, since living here—most everybody here is from Africa or from India—I've become less intolerant.*
>
> *Researcher:* Interesting. Why do you think that is?
>
> *Mr. Braskey: I recognize…they've got the same sense of humor. They like, they love, they laugh, they cry, they get attached.…And hey, they treat me great. I don't know why—but they say I'm one of their pets.*

Although in the past Mr. Braskey would—based on his own description—have been angry or uncomfortable, or otherwise have had a poor quality experience due to his forced exposure to people of other races, this change in his attitude permitted him to have a much higher quality experience with the care staff at Wetherby Place.

Although changes in resident health and functioning have been the primary focus in shaping state AL policies and in daily AL operations, bringing forward the changes in AL settings is also essential to understanding the shifting quality balance between person and place through time. Consequently, it is important to view changes in residents as inclusive of a broader array of both subtle and major changes occurring in their lives, including positive ones, that are likely to influence their evaluations of quality. Given the established focus on resident health decline, much of the remainder of this chapter focuses on how dynamics of place (ALs as places to live, work, visit, and receive care) can shift subtly or dramatically over the course of weeks, months, or years.

CHANGES IN THE AL SETTING

Ownership Change

During our research, ownership of some AL sites changed. Ownership transitions may cause major shifts in quality, potentially influencing the philosophy of care, available services, the target client base, and the cost of care, as well as staff size, composition, or performance. One clear example of a dramatic change was at Murray Ridge, where our initial contact was with its founder, Mr. Hill. As a modest-sized, family-owned AL, Mr. Hill had converted a nursing home building to AL and was actively engaged with the provider network for the state. He held clear ideas of what AL's niche should be and emphasized support of his limited but loyal staff to ensure that they could meet resident needs. In fact, he was quite attentive to staff needs, given that residents come and go, but staff members (hopefully) stay for a long time; many of his staff had been there for many years. Mr. Hill also bent general rules as he saw fit in order to best serve individual residents and their families. If staff shortages or emergencies arose, he was equally likely to either fix the plumbing or to undertake resident care himself, over and above his management duties. His assistant, Darlene Hall, was like many other staff, having come to work there as a teenaged relative of another staffer. She had worked her way up to the associate director slot when, unexpectedly, Mr. Hill died.

The Hill family decided to continue operation of Murray Ridge, hiring an experienced nursing home administrator, Clarice Watson, to undertake its daily management. Ms. Watson, however, brought different ideas to running Murray Ridge, which altered daily life and routines and upset many. Residents and staff alike said it seemed much more like a nursing home than when under Mr. Hill's leadership. During her tenure, some residents and staff members became sufficiently dissatisfied to "vote with their feet," displeased with Ms. Watson's "nursing home" approach to AL. When it became clear that this arrangement was not working, the family hired a familiar person, Janice Pugh, to return Murray Ridge to its prior philosophy and routine. Ms. Pugh restored many of the old rules of everyday life for residents and staff alike, but also left after an unsuccessful attempt to purchase Murray Ridge. This led to Darlene's promotion as executive director at the relatively young age of 28. Clearly, the change in leadership was disruptive, resulting in departures of both staff and residents before the facility returned to equilibrium. Darlene was uniquely positioned to provide continuity, given her years of experience there. However, not all ownership transitions are equally influential.

Another of our settings, Winter Hills, had been independently owned during its initial seven years of operation. It was remarkable for the majority of staff, who had been there for those full seven years. A chain purchased Winter Hills during our study, raising the question of whether daily life or staff and services might change there. Other than some expansion of the marketing of Winter Hills, it appears that local leadership, staff, and residents have mostly remained in place, with daily life little altered from before the ownership shift. In short, although changing ownership does not guarantee that other changes will follow, it provides the potential for key aspects relating to AL quality to shift.

Ms. Lovedahl, a resident complained in her interview about the negative impact of new ownership at the Greenbriar. The new company had, according to her account, reduced the number of care staff from three to two per shift. Her daughter had complained that, if anyone was ill, especially on weekends, it would be problematic, because there might be only one care provider at Greenbriar for all its residents. In a fourth setting that we studied, multiple rounds of ownership change prompted frequent leadership turnover, with residents and staff having to repeatedly learn to adapt to different leadership styles and priorities.

AL Managers: Change in Leadership

Residents often voiced their views on the quality or style of leadership exercised by AL management, particularly on the executive director or other top managers. Watching as leaders came and went, sometimes in rapid succession, provided an opportunity for residents to compare how everyday life and quality changed following a shift in the AL's director. Residents' responses to leadership varied, from the (sometimes grudging) acceptance of the authority of the Sisters running St. Brigid AL to a more critical analysis of the business and "people skills" of corporately appointed leaders. New managers often brought with them differing philosophies about AL, which altered important aspects of services in the setting or in how daily life unfolded.

Alan Cohen at Wetherby Place had, after several years in residence there, seen many changes, including major building renovations, an increase in the proportion of residents with dementia, and multiple turnovers in the executive director position, for a variety of reasons. Mr. Cohen linked changes in his evaluation of quality to these leadership changes.

Mr. Cohen: Well, for one thing he [current executive director]—let's put it this way, of all the directors, there was one lady who was a woman director, she was very good. She ran this place right. But she got sick and she couldn't continue, so they had to appoint other directors, and they didn't function as well as she did. But this current one—I think they could have appointed him maybe a month or two ago—he's as good as she was.

Researcher: Oh, yeah?

Mr. Cohen: He sees to things that haven't been done before and he does them and he's open to residents to talk to, so he's pretty good. . . .

Researcher: When you say he's as good as the woman before him. . . what things are good about what. . . he does?

Mr. Cohen: Well, for one thing they made sure that our needs are taken care of. They're always open to us if we complain or if we want to put in suggestions, they're all ears, and she was open to us and that's very good. I mean residents should be able to do that. And that's what I consider good.

Ms. Meisel said that the hiring of a new nurse was perhaps the first of a series of changes of key staff at Boxwood Gardens as new corporate ownership took hold. *"It's all changing over. The new corporate headquarters sent a new person in. . . .who knows what [the new nurse will] be like—she's young."* Such transitions led to periods of learning how best to work with a new leadership within the AL—whether they made themselves available in public areas for regular conversations and feedback or remained cloistered in the office all day, were open to new ideas or set in their goals, and if they focused more on the residents' needs or on their corporate bosses' goals and priorities.

In contrast to Mr. Cohen's experience, Dr. Styles indicated that an ownership change for the Greenbriar was not disruptive in his view.

Dr. Styles: They've changed management [ownership], but they still have the same people, basically the same people running this operation. But it's part of a large national chain and that management has changed.

Researcher: So the people that you've been working with here are still caring and all those kind of things.

Dr. Styles: Yes, they're basically the same people. The person who was the acting director when I first came over here is no longer here. She was a registered nurse and the director of nursing here when the regular director went on maternity leave. She was pretty capable I thought and got along well. She's no longer here but she's got a better job but doing much the same thing, I suppose at another place. But by and large the people who were the managers of this and that or the other things are still here.

Several residents mentioned dissatisfaction with new directors who stayed in their offices all day, unaware of happenings on the floors with the residents, with their mid-level managers, or with direct care staff. In some instances, problems of leadership were attributed to the decisions of "corporate bosses." According to Martha St. John, this was the case at Boxwood Gardens, as the AL's mission was shifted toward people requiring more care than had previously been the case.

[I]f you are taking more [residents in] on that level that require more care—which means that you require more assistants, more nurse's aides...when they're all like that. And then—and they run into a labor problem. You have—mostly a staff by green card labor....[W]hen I first came here the head of nursing was from Nigeria and then they didn't have a nursing director, they didn't have an executive director and they didn't have a marketing director.... That's, I think, corporate's idea. They just had the lease. [Then] they hired an executive director and a nursing director and both of them...were very well trained....but I think it was corporate's idea [that] there would be a minority [of needed staff in place] and they were women, so I think they could bring them up to do the corporate's ideas.... So after about 4 or 5 months they left. Nothing was ever said, but I think that was it. So then they got somebody that filled in. And...that one guy...he was really quite good at taking over, but he had the courage to quit right then and there, and he said, no, I can't operate this way [without enough staff]. So, our corporate—I don't know if they learned or not....

And they have a continual training problem—orientation. I say, when somebody's really different [good], why don't you give them a raise and keep them? To me that would be cheaper.

Clearly a number of settings had leadership changes, with some residents attributing notable changes in quality to turnover in these key positions.

Staffing Issues

Staff size, training, and performance are issues often evaluated in AL settings' own consumer satisfaction studies, and may also be a focus in states' AL regulations. Size and training of the care staff are items that are more easily measured in a survey; staff attitudes, performance, and retention are also commonly discussed as central challenges to AL administrators or owners (Ball, Perkins, Hollingsworth, & Kemp, 2010; Hodlewsky, 2001; Stearns, Zimmerman, & Park, 2004). Having sufficient staff and having the right mix of training and professional preparation is a necessary basic ingredient to quality; our focus here is on how staff changes influence the shifting quality balance between residents' needs and preferences and what the AL setting is able to deliver (see Chapter 3 for a focus on other aspects of care).

Most of the AL managers or executive directors we interviewed pointed out the challenges of getting and keeping a good staff, well motivated for this work. Directors mentioned the efforts they undertook to ensure that they had the staff necessary to conduct the essential tasks of daily life in AL. Both Tina Giles (Boxwood Gardens) and Samuel Meadows (Wetherby Place) indicated the importance of this quality. Meadows said,

> We try to work with everybody [staff] as much as we can, because...[t]here is a very small pool to choose from. And we try to work with anybody that we bring on board.... We lose people for economics, we lose people for education, career advancement—so our turnover, I think is probably less than 10% a year.... [I]f you don't have the staff, you can't take care of the people. Even though our staffing is good you still have vacations, sick [days], daily life to deal with.... [K]eeping up that [resident] census and then, when the census goes low, getting your census back up so you can keep your staff happy, so you don't have to cut the staff's hours, which in turn keeps the [residents] happy.

Tina Giles said that she walked into a "skeleton crew" of workers when she arrived, due to staff attrition. A major task for her was to rebuild and stabilize the staff by establishing a constructive relationship with them.

I think they understand what your expectations are and you recognize them and you appreciate them for what they do. I think the recognition piece is a big piece. Our turnover has definitely started to drop.... once you sort of lay your groundwork...you hold them accountable.... [W]e...have a pretty good group.... We have some really good ones that have been in nursing school [and] they're excellent.... Dependable, phenomenal with the residents, great on assessments. They're all about the resident care and getting their job done and managing the staff that's with them when they're around.

The religiously sponsored St. Brigid had a mixture of long-time workers and a cadre subject to turnover due to poor motivation, absenteeism or tardiness, or competition from better jobs, according to its director, Sister Barbara.

> *Researcher:* Do you have any challenges with staffing?
>
> *Sister Barbara:* Oh yes. There's always a little circular door that goes around for the ones that come in—but it's few. I'd say more than half of our employees are here from anywhere from 36, 38 years. A good many of them 20 or 25, a good many of them 15. There's that little percentage, you know that keep using the revolving door. [laughs]...No one stays here that really doesn't have a love for what they're doing, health care, they don't stay. Anybody that's unkind, or uses bad words—they don't stay, because they can tell they're out of place. We don't keep them.... We're very strict with tardiness and absenteeism; some of our best people cannot stay because they're tardy.... [W]e can't compete with hospitals, we really can't. So that if one of our very good nurses gets an offer, she's an LPN and they'll pay for her education to become an RN, well naturally you know we have to say well, we can't do that. We know it and wish you well.

Joyce Henderson said that Arcadia Springs faced a challenge, particularly in keeping part-time workers, but that they had one advantage missing at many other settings.

> [A] lot of these young ladies unfortunately, at the salaries that we have to pay them, can't afford cars. It gets to be cost prohibitive for them, or they have old cars, which I drive too, but that break down.... [W]e're on the bus line. I can't tell you how many times

I've had people come to me, and come here and say that they left other jobs that paid more and will take our job because we're right on the bus line....My staffing turnover for my part-timers is like 60%. That's high, OK, but my staffing turnover for most of my staff that are permanent is only like 13%. So we've got a lot of people who have been here 3, 4, 5 years.

Issues of staffing and staff turnover were widely discussed by residents in interviews. Both the number of staff and the presence of particularly qualified or skilled staff in key areas were mentioned regularly. According to Ms. Pollock, this situation is subject of dark humor at Boxwood Gardens. When asked if staff turnover is high, she said, *"There is. The joke around here, and it's not very funny, [is that] another ship [a new staff person] just came in. But it's true."* Ms. Carson was very vocal about the staff's limitations in training, being from other cultures, and the high rate of turnover. She identified two *"infamous phrases"* she heard regularly from staff. They were *"I'll be back,"* meaning that a resident will never see the staffer again when she still needs help, and *"You're not on my list tonight."* According to fieldnotes of this discussion with Ms. Carson, she *"would like to see staff regularly come so that every resident gets to know four or five staff members really well, and staff members could better serve residents if they were more familiar with them,"* expressing (knowingly or not) a tenet of the Culture Change movement (Thomas, 2004). As to daily encounters with staff, Ms. Carson said *"They're in a rush—and they rush in and rush out. I'm trying to talk to them, they're already out the door and halfway down the hall, and I'm talking to myself. They have no time."*

Peter Granier, a resident, reinforced the importance of staffing levels for his life at the Greenbriar. When asked what he would make a priority if he was in charge there, he said,

I would try to make sure that they don't have big turnover in the workers here, in the help. It seems like they get some good people and the next thing you know, they're out and for some reason or other nobody knows why. They say oh, she resigned, or he resigned.

Researcher: They don't give you any feedback or...Why do you think that the staff leaves?

Mr. Granier: There's been a big changeover since I've been here. I've been here about two and half years now—there's been a big change since then.

Mr. Leland at St. Brigid highlighted what might have seemed a very minor staff change that influenced his quality in the area of meals.

They had a lady that takes care of the lunchroom where we have our meals and...when I came, she was there all the time. When I say all the time—there's two people. There's one that takes care of breakfast and lunch and then one for dinner.... But she was on the first two meals—in here every day, and she was good. She left and since she's gone, they haven't worked anything out well.

Rather than replacing the dining room supervisor, the sisters running St. Brigid attempted to cover that work using other staff, who did not perform the job as well, because it was an "extra duty."

Ms. McCoy told us that the activities weren't good anymore at Arcadia Springs because a former activities director left.

I really think that it's [pause] below my capabilities, let's put it that way. There are some people that it's fine for, and there are other people that it's like, "Whoa, excuse me!" You feel, like I said, like a little kid about that big [gesturing]—you know? When I first came in here there was another woman, Cassie—I don't know her last name. But she made things fun. She didn't put you down. She didn't say anything negative about anybody, no matter who it was. And she was to me a good [activities director].

Jill Kates reflected upon problems beyond turnover, noting the poor attitudes of staff at Wetherby Place, over and above her concerns about the language barrier with Spanish-speaking staff.

Ms. Kates: [T]his place—they have more people working that I haven't even seen before. I don't know why. You know all the time I'm looking at this woman—I haven't seen her before. Why always hiring? I don't know.

Researcher: Do you think people are quitting and they're replacing them, or are they just adding on?

Ms. Kates: They're adding.... and then some of them... some of them are kind of—well, they're like sarcastic. If you ask for something, there's sarcasm. Well, not with me, because they wouldn't get away with it. There's a couple of them that I would like to see them gone, I really would. They don't belong with people like me.

Many residents identified low pay as an issue in staff turnover and recognized the fiscal constraints that limited the size, composition, and quality of staff. Ms. Rosenstein felt short-changed by having no activity staff during the weekends, saying *"They forget about us. They don't care."* She was told she could run the exercise activity herself using a taped exercise routine, but limited staffing also caused problems in finding someone to retrieve and set up the tape recorder.

> *So instead of starting at 9:30, we'll start...after 10:00. And I'm one...who's right on time. And it's boring—you sit there and wait. That's the trouble here—we wait, and wait. You get to learn patience. But we sit and wait for everything....Nothing's on time.*

Not all resident and management views of staff and staff turnover were negative. Many residents noted how hardworking and caring staff members were in attending to details and personalizing their daily care. Mr. Dugan permitted staff members at Greenbriar to take breaks in his room. *"[L]et them come in, let them rest a little bit. Because I don't think they're paid enough to begin with. I think they get—I don't know what they get paid, but it's low."* Mrs. Grier of St. Brigid cried and couldn't sleep when she learned that a favorite staff member, whom she and her husband thought of as an adopted daughter, was being fired for being repeatedly late to work. They were secretly planning strategies to keep in touch with her in the future, because she'd been special to them. Mildred Ashman noted the friendliness and hard work of the care staff at Wetherby Place,

> *They're very friendly that way. And there are certain nurse's aides that—Lord knows—if she's here for the night, then I'll be put to bed. In the evening if my aide—I don't have a permanent one, but the one that takes care of me most of the time—if she's not here, there are three or four that will come in to see if I'm wanting to go to bed. They're real good that way, filling in for each other.*

Dr. Luckinbill, a resident at Wetherby Place, said at the start of his interview that he invited the new staff members, mostly African immigrants, who came into his room to work to take the time to point out on a map their countries of origin. He expressed interest in their cultures, in contrast to the disdain expressed by others with regard to immigrants working in AL settings.

Tina Giles said that not all turnover at Boxwood Gardens came about for negative reasons, noting the number of staff who were seeking further education to advance in the field.

> *Tina:* You know this industry, it turns over. I can't say I've been anywhere, where I hadn't had a turnover—especially with nurses. [I]f I get a nurse that stays two years, that's a plus—that's like forever for them. You look at the résumés that come in. Some of them don't even put the month anymore, because they just put the year, because...sometimes it's 9 months, 10 months....And then you have growth. We have some of these CNAs [Certified Nurses Assistants] that are in school now for LPN [Licensed Practical Nurse program]....
>
> *Researcher:* So you do see them moving on?
>
> *Tina:* Oh, yeah—quite a few. Quite a few.

Family members also informed us that combinations of changes in leadership and staff influenced their perceptions of quality, changing their entire sense of an AL over time. Alice and Don Waltrip referred to such changes at Arcadia Springs during Alice's mother's stay there, comparing their first impression upon visiting with more recent conditions.

> *Alice:* Oh, the first time—well, the woman Cassie isn't there any longer. She was wonderful. She was wonderful with the patients and she's the one that talked to me at the time. She was also the PR person, and since [then] she had moved on to just doing the activities. But she explained everything, and she was very good. She was good at selling stuff, you know.
>
> *Researcher:* Has a nice personality.
>
> *Alice:* And the place was so clean at the time and the people seemed content. You know it was nice they could go out on the front porch and they said, yeah, we'll take your Mom out on the porch, and blah, blah, blah, blah. So, that was my...
>
> *Don:* It was very nice. It was clean—you walked in—
>
> *Alice:* It always smelled...clean, which I always figured wouldn't be the case and isn't the case now....
>
> *Don:* And the rooms were real nice and we looked at some of the ones where people lived and at the time they had

people—husbands and wives that lived there that actually had cars and would come and go. So it wasn't as if they were confined there, like a nursing home. So it just seemed real pleasant. Real homey, I guess.

[Comparing to recent times]

Don: I mean you know as far as the clothing, and as far as the cleanliness and the hygiene and all the other little things that they mention [as services], they don't exist. I mean it just doesn't happen. But sometimes we walk in there and you just see where there's stuff all over the rugs or the place smells like urine. . . .

Given these changes, the couple said it bothered them to pay the full amount. But they knew if they withheld part of their payment, "They'd move you out of there real quick."

ALs in the Larger Economy

AL settings are also influenced by the larger context of the community marketplaces in which they operate, as well as by trends in the larger economy. Whereas residents sometimes noted that an AL had shifted its focus or marketing toward a particular niche, executive directors were particularly aware of these larger dynamics as influences on the quality balance. Joyce Henderson, director of Arcadia Springs, addressed the basic economic dynamic she encountered.

There's no such thing as stable in assisted living. I don't think anybody's census is hardly ever stable. And most people who tell you that—you talk to the Administrator off the record, they're lying. There are very few places where it's really stable. Assisted living goes through these huge ebbs and tides and a lot of it we try to figure out. I try to look at what's going on in the financial market and get a feel for what's happening, because a lot of has to do with basically [being] private pay driven, what or how the economy is feeling at the time. Because, if people are feeling good, like they have the money, well sure we can put Mom there and let her spend her money and that will take care of her, and this that and the other. But if they're anxious about their own financial stability, they may

start to think about that inheritance that Mom's got and not want
her to give that money up.

Tina Giles recognized the change in recent years, as people came to
visit the AL in more of a crisis situation, in part due to the difficulty of
selling a home or financing care in a time of economic stress.

> *Researcher:* Do you find residents coming into assisted living more
> frail?
>
> *Tina Giles:* Oh, most definitely. They're staying at home a lot
> longer. The families are keeping them, trying to put support
> services in place; they're trying to do it themselves a lot longer.
> The...residents aren't telling them of their ailments and the things
> that are happening, you know, so that they're there unsafe a lot
> longer. And usually when a person comes in, a lot of times it's a
> crisis, you know. And that's one of the first questions we ask—you
> know, what brought you to us today? "Mom fell yesterday." Come
> to find out she hadn't been taking her medicine and her pills hadn't
> been refilled, you know, the refrigerator had everything in it was
> moldy, that kind of thing. Or they had a fall, so they ended up in
> the hospital, and that's when they went to the hospital and...they
> realized the condition.

Other directors focused on their immediate competition in their
local areas, even including other ALs of the same chain. Two directors
who were interviewed indicated that their ALs, while not providing
the most amenities, offered other things that residents valued, thereby
filling an important slot in the AL market. Tina Giles was very aware
of her competition and how Boxwood Gardens compared to other
providers in the area, including the differences in the clientele they
attracted.

> *Researcher:* You mentioned that you think that this location is a
> negative?
>
> *Tina:* Well, not necessarily a negative but we don't get half...[the]
> people coming through [compared to competitors]. You know,
> we're so close to [nearby AL of the same chain] and so close to
> [another AL] that there are three of us right here together. And so
> it's not—we don't have the same traffic that the other buildings

have. We have a lot of little small, you know, even if it's Mom and Pop, you know, assisted livings right around the corner from us, which makes it really difficult to compete. So yes, we're in a kind of quirk, so we have to find what our niche is here and focus on that, and just focus on doing that really well.

Researcher: Can you characterize the people who live here?

Tina: It's tough—oh boy, we have such a mixture. But I guess I'd say the underlying basis of our residents—we have a very, what's the word I want to use—this is a family-oriented facility, I should say. If you walk in some of—I can always give you examples from some of our other buildings. The residents here—the [nearby chain partner] building doesn't necessarily appeal to them, because it's you know—the lavish, the marble floors, the grand chandelier when you walk through the front door. They're homey—I call them [residents at Boxwood Gardens] home bodies, as we all are. You know, company—they want the chair out front with the foot cushion where they can sit there and lounge in the lobby. You know, you'll notice—you go into other buildings you won't see the same. It's totally different from ours.... These are the residents, I would say, they were either quite a few homemakers, you know worked for a while, retired, will have spent their time just raising their family, or their grand- children.... or just like they spent a lot of time at home. You know, you have the residents that took care of the flowers, you know the garden.

Similarly, Joyce Henderson identified the particular strengths of Arcadia Springs, relative to its immediate competition. When asked how it compared, she said,

... It's more affordable, and it's more of the lifestyle that somebody who wants to—who has been used to living a nice middle class life. They're not looking for maid service, they're not looking for three star china restaurant, because if they are then we're not going to suit them. There are other places out there that have all of that. But if you want somebody who truly cares about you, who truly is going to watch over you, who's going to make sure you get the things you need and know who you are, and know what your likes are and who your family are when they call, then this is more the place.

The Changing Social Context of Other Residents

As a result of economic dynamics and other external forces influencing the operation of ALs, decisions about admission and retention of residents changed (and continue to change) during our research, resulting in modified profiles of people residing there. New residents who became part of the social context of everyday life for their peers, as well as the aging in place of longer-term residents with the likelihood of cognitive or physical decline, reshaped everyday life for everyone in the setting. In particular, these changes influenced the social dimensions of daily events, such as meals or activities, where groups of residents share a physical space and social experience.

Change in the profile of residents being served in an AL setting also frequently meant increased demand on limited staff energies. Consequently, differences among new residents and changes for continuing residents sometimes raised quality concerns. For example, Mrs. Wyler, who had lived for some time at Boxwood Gardens when we interviewed her, noticed changes as the AL had attempted to carve out a distinct identity caring for older adults with cognitive issues. She said,

> When I came here, I don't know how many, but there were not nearly so many mental patients as there are [now]. And now it's written up that way. It's not just Boxwood Gardens for Assisted Living....and Mental— that's on the [sign], that's outside on the gate I think.

The change in focus, and the shifting balance toward residents with dementia, altered the social environment and the activities of Boxwood Gardens in an undesirable direction, toward lower quality, in her view.

Aside from such purposeful shifts, the regular processes of aging in place and resident turnover gradually alter the profile of people sharing everyday life in AL. In interviews, residents commented a good deal about the similarities or differences among people living in their ALs. Primary among the comments were those relating to the cognitive and physical functioning of their peers. Other traits that mattered to at least some residents of AL included those typical of any community, such as religion, gender, and age, all of which still mattered to those living in the social context of AL.

Turning first to cognitive problems, the poor cognitive state of other residents at Wetherby Place frustrated Fred Braskey's wish to get a group together to play bridge. He complained that [he], *"Can't get a bridge game going. Can't get the players....All of them love to play bridge, but they've forgotten how to play it. So, it's very difficult to get bridge players together."* Other residents used stigmatizing terms like *"vegetable"* or *"mental patient"* to describe those sharing the public spaces, activities, and meals with them in AL. Martha St. John described herself as *"in the minority"* at Boxwood Gardens, because she was reasonably healthy and cognitively intact, aspects that had changed over time in those around her. Activities were no longer of interest to her, because they were *"...down to the lowest common denominator,"* serving the majority there with limited cognitive function. Ms. Wyler admitted that she hadn't made many friends at Boxwood Gardens because of most people's limited cognition. The few friends she's made are *"mainly with the ones who are still able to think. The others I talk to—you know some of them, it would be no use to try to make friends with. But those who are able, yeah."* Lorraine Heilbrun missed the social side of her daily routines at Wetherby Place, including casual conversation.

> *I don't need craftwork. I'd like discussions on what goes on in the world; [that] is what I'm looking for. Or just discussing where you've been in the world or what you've seen, or what you saw on TV. I mean I do talk to the man at my table who is a former principal....and we can talk about what's going on, on TV with the politics and all and that's all I'm looking for. I'm not looking for a discussion at a very high level; it's a normal social kind of thing.*

Physical challenges of others, and consequent limitations in their capacity and interest in being active and engaged, were source of consternation to some residents. Mr. Levenson prepared a lecture on big band music, one of his lifetime interests, for others at Wetherby Place. He said that when the event finally came, *"nine people showed up, five of them slept."* Feeling his time had been wasted, he vowed never to devote so much effort again to an activity there. Ms. Kates echoed Mr. Levenson's concerns about others' disinterest.

> *And like I'm saying—the people here are not active at all. I mean, you've only maybe got two people that do things, but the rest of the people— forget it. You know they just don't bother. So I spend most of my time watching my TV.*

Later she added, "...Probably if my mind was gone it wouldn't bother me."

Ms. Meisel was distressed by encountering others with health problems and limited cognitive capacities on a daily basis at Boxwood Gardens.

> The conversations are so miniscule because so many of them are so sickly and, I mean, they've been cogged over, they had strokes, they eat with their fingers, they have to be pampered like little babies to eat. There are so many depressing issues—it's really not pleasurable for me to be even at the same table with them. I can't begin to tell you the dissipation I have.

Martha St. John, having grown comfortable at her AL, had earlier regretted not having chosen one of several area senior communities for independent living and noted that her AL's clientele had changed over time.

> I remember when I first moved in here, and I was talking to the marketing people. I said, I don't mean this the way it sounds and I don't really know what I expected, maybe something like [names large CCRC]. But I didn't expect to find so many handicapped people. And it was really very—I said, oh there's a wheelchair. And it was so erratic. I mean all combinations of dementia, you know and forgetfulness and sometimes—they could come out with something so astounding, it was—I mean it was very—and it took me a long time to, well, finally I adjusted to that and I discovered that I am in a minority.

Continuing this topic later, she said, "I suppose I would...like to have not so many, what I would call invalids. I would like to have it more a half and half rather than being in the minority."

Clearly the changes over time in both the physical health and cognitive functioning of their peers challenge quality views of residents. ALs serving mixed clientele by including those with dementia in the general setting, rather than in a special care unit, as was the case in most of our study sites, faced—daily—the challenge of accommodating the diverse needs of high functioning people and those whose cognition is failing. But, in addition, the presence or absence of people who share a similar social background was mentioned with some regularity in resident interviews as influencing quality and the sense of community.

Ms. Strauss missed the companionship of those who shared her faith. When asked what she liked about Murray Ridge, she suggested it would be better, *"if I had a few more of my kind... like Baptists, my beliefs."* In contrast, Margaret Dressler, living in a Catholic-sponsored setting, noted that religious differences were less problematic than she expected. *"I knew Catholics, yeah. But I'm Baptist and I have to say the Catholic people are pretty good people. They're just as good as the Baptist."* Ms. Pollock was surprised to find both a regular Mass and many other Catholics living at Boxwood Gardens. *"Well, what surprised me is—[the] first time they were a little late [starting Mass] and I just sat there looking around... I counted 45 Catholics—residents. And this surprised me, but about everyone I sit with says they're Catholic."*

Several men and women mentioned the gender imbalance typical of AL populations. Perry Sluchak would *"like to see a couple more good men.... [who] would see life like I do,"* at Murray Ridge, and Mr. Leland easily listed the names of the three other males residing with him at St. Brigid. In contrast, Ms. Powell was dismayed that there were any men *at all* residing at St. Brigid, and had developed a feud with one of them that played itself out in insulting verbal exchanges in the dining room. While we saw both cross-sex friendships and some segregation of the sexes in dining and events, Mr. Wayne at the Greenbriar found the affinity at his table in the dining room welcome, noting that men at his dinner table, *"...most are retired people, military, so we've got things in common."*

Another dimension of difference identified by residents was age, with some interviewees expressing ageism. Anna Ames of the Greenbriar, who was younger than most people living there, said, for example,

> The people here are older and they don't talk much. They mostly read or they're doing some kind of activity. They listen a lot—people come in and read to them in some way or another. The church comes in and there are seminars and services and stuff, so basically and we play things like bingo and Pokeno...

She felt disconnected, because their orientations and interests differed from her own. A stronger view came from Ms. Rosenstein at Wetherby Place. *"I don't see anybody here that I would want to* associate with. All they talk about is their illness and their families, or their grandchildren. I have grandchildren, but I don't talk about them." She said instead she'd prefer conversations about "Books and everyday things going on." When the researcher asked Ms. Salguiero, who referred to some residents as "vegetables," where she got her hair done, she said that she colors it herself, "every once in a while.... I don't want my hair to turn white, not yet." When asked why, she replied, "I just don't... All their hair is white" [speaking of others who live there]. According to the interview notes, Ms. Salguiero expressed her disdain for other residents, implying that gray hair meant that they had all "given up."

QUALITY AS A PROCESS, NOT A PRODUCT

This chapter has addressed a dynamic that is key to understanding changes in resident quality in AL—the fact that many elements of both the resident-evaluator and of the AL that influence quality are subject to change through time. Beyond pragmatics of price and location, part of the process of selecting an AL setting for oneself, a friend, or relative is to seek the best possible balance between the person's life experiences, current needs, and preferences and the offerings of an AL. This balance, however, is likely to shift if the resident ages in place for a substantial period of time. In some instances, these changes may actually improve the alignment between person and setting, leading to higher quality and greater satisfaction. It is also possible, however, if there was a good initial match with the AL, that resident satisfaction may be diminished as he or she changes, the AL setting changes, or both change.

Although residents' declining health and cognitive decline have been widely recognized as influential in both quality assessment and in leading to transitions, other types of resident changes, which may reshape their profiles of experiences, needs, and preferences, have largely been neglected. In particular, improvements in health or functioning, and changes in attitudes or perceptions about life in AL, which might enhance the fit between person and place and improve quality, have not been recognized. Changes within the resident, particularly those that alter her needs or preferences, may diminish her alignment with the physical, social, or service environment of a particular AL setting.

Importantly, the multiple types of change that happen to AL settings, with the exception of staff size or turnover, have remained largely unexamined. These AL-level changes may have little or no impact on certain residents, due to their varying priorities and expectations, but may result in either improvement or erosion of quality assessments for others. As we have seen, changes to an AL setting, including ownership change, leadership (and philosophy) change, alterations in the staffing levels or orientation, as well as changes in the profile of the overall resident population, may alter how residents evaluate their AL experience. Although most concern naturally focuses on things that diminish quality, it also is possible for change in the person or in the place they live to improve the balance between resident and AL, resulting in improvement in quality ratings by a resident.

Daily events in the AL provide opportunities for ongoing reevaluation of quality. Encounters of residents with staff, services (personal care, meals, or activities), the physical environment, and the other residents (individually or collectively) have the potential to reshape an individual's quality evaluation on any given day. A caregiver who forgets to return to assist someone left on the toilet, another who takes extra time to personalize clothing choices in the morning or to make sure that the soup is served hot, or a run-in with another resident over seating in the dining room may all influence certain individuals' evaluations of quality in a positive or negative direction. For other residents, these particular events might be dismissed or go unnoticed, but a change in management or a gradual move toward focusing on dementia care might be influential on their quality views. Therefore, quality is not only an ever-changing balance, but it is also an individualized process, with distinctive priorities for each quality evaluator.

Few settings we have studied remained stable in personnel, leadership, services, and so on, over months or years; the degree of stability at Winter Hills, discussed earlier in this chapter, is relatively rare. The ongoing changes that occur with routine turnover of staff and residents can easily modify the climate and daily routines of an AL in important ways that have an impact on quality—and, even if the setting remains stable, residents are experiencing changes, including those in their functioning and preferences, which may diminish the balance between that person and that AL through time.

There are, of course, a variety of potential responses to any diminished quality that results from changes over time within AL settings. Theoretically, as a consumer-based sector, dissatisfied residents would simply move to another setting that is in better balance with their needs and preferences. However, only a few residents or families we spoke to welcomed the idea of moving, preferring to stay and make it work in the current setting if possible. The consumer approach also is mismatched with the suggestion that is often made to accept a particular AL as one's home—people only reluctantly walk away from someplace they feel to be home.

As a result of these multilayered dynamics, everyone living or working in AL is constantly adapting to changes, which make the achievement of quality a moving target, a constant shifting of the quality balance for any individual. For example, continuing to meet the activity needs of a minority of residents who are cognitively able, as the needs of their cognitively impaired peers change, seems to require scheduling separate sets of activities, a feat that is challenging on a limited budget. Consequently, emphasis may shift toward serving the majority, leaving those who are higher-functioning with few satisfying activities. Individuals who arrive with good physical functioning may come to appreciate care staff more, or may experience increased frustration as their reliance on others for daily care and mobility assistance grows. Residents (or family members) who evaluate the AL as a health care setting, employing the medical model, may prioritize those issues, either due to the resident's need for substantial care and services or based on their understanding of AL's role as primarily medical. For other residents, however, the role of AL is to reduce daily demands for cooking and cleaning, as well as to provide opportunities for socializing. Clearly, excelling in both of these somewhat contradictory roles is challenging to owners, managers, and staff members. Consequently, change and the need to adapt to change are constant challenges for those operating or working in AL settings, particularly those intent to provide high-quality, personalized care.

REFERENCES

Ball, M. M., Perkins, M. M., Hollingsworth, C., & Kemp, C. L. (2010). *Frontline workers in assisted living.* Baltimore, MD: Johns Hopkins University Press.

Eckert, J. K., Carder, P. C., Morgan, L. A., Frankowski, A. C., & Roth, E. G. (2009). *Inside assisted living: The search for home.* Baltimore, MD: Johns Hopkins University Press.

Hodlewsky, R. T. (2001). Staffing problems and strategies in assisted living. In S. I. Zimmerman, P. Sloane, & J. K. Eckert (Eds.), *Assisted living: Needs, practices and policies in residential care for the elderly.* Baltimore, MD: Johns Hopkins University Press.

Stearns, S., Zimmerman, S., & Park, J. (2004). Determinants and effects of staffing mix and intensity in residential care/assisted living. *The Gerontologist, 44,* 247–248.

Thomas, W. H. (2004). *What are old people for? How older people will save the world.* Acton, MA: VanderWyk and Burnham.

Wolinsky, F., Callahan, C., Fitzgerald, F., & Johnson, R. (1993). Changes in functional status and the risks of subsequent nursing home placement and death. *Journal of Gerontology: Social Sciences, 48*(3), S94–101.

8
Moving Toward Quality Balance
Lessons Learned From Residents

Reflecting on the material presented in the earlier chapters of this book, a seminal lesson to be learned is that conveyed by Ms. Gentile, a resident of Boxwood Gardens:

> *Researcher:* If someone you knew was moving into assisted living…what would you suggest that she look for in finding a place?
>
> *Ms. Gentile: The first thing you have to do is know in your mind and in your heart you can do this…don't come in expecting all your cares and worries to end. They won't. You have to come in with an open mind and a heart that's open to give. But there's no panacea to any of it. What you look for is, what can you live with, because it's up here [points to head] and in here [points to heart]. If you can't handle that, you're in a heap of trouble. You have to know that you can do this. You have to make up your mind.*
>
> *Researcher:* When you came looking at Boxwood Gardens, what were some of the things that you were looking at and what you were thinking about when you came?
>
> *Ms. Gentile: Well, my children and I talked about it. One wanted me in Ohio, one wanted me in Florida—but that meant new doctors, new places, and I wasn't that adjustable. I'm familiar with my surroundings here. The neighborhood, the community—I grew up here with my family and so it was what I was looking for: peace of mind.*
>
> *Researcher:* What would you tell your neighbor who was looking, what would you tell her to make sure that she avoided in selecting a place?
>
> *Ms. Gentile: Expecting everything to be better for them. Expecting to be waited on hand and foot, kowtowed to, if you will. You have to put forth some effort.*

This advice, in the context of what has been presented in earlier chapters, draws our attention to one of the more interesting aspects related to considering the quality of assisted living (AL): most residents, families, and the public in general have expectations about AL. These expectations may be positive or negative, and may put uneven responsibility for the quality balance on either themselves or on the AL provider. Residents with unrealistically high expectations may have been swayed by influential marketing or encouraging children, or may have difficulty accepting the limitations of their own conditions; these may be the residents for whom achieving the quality balance will be more challenging. A related inherent challenge is that those "expecting to be waited on hand and foot, kowtowed to, if you will" may suffer if the environment robs them of the necessity to attend to their own needs as much as they are able. The phenomenon of "learned helplessness" was originally understood as an individual's reaction when he or she could not control the outcome of a situation (Seligman, 1975), but one also may learn to be helpless if the environment presents no demands (Lawton & Nahemow, 1975). Thus, moving toward quality balance is important not only for peaceful relations but also for physical and mental well-being.

The points listed earlier are not intended to convey that most residents had unrealistic expectations in terms of quality in AL, or to suggest that providers are naive about the needs and wants of residents. Indeed, much of what we heard from residents earlier in the book is likely to be familiar to providers, including understanding that frames of reference, expectations, and service needs are diverse. What may be less familiar, however, are those different perspectives of quality seen in a practical manner, and how they translate to actions that providers and others can take to maximize and promote quality before, during, and after a resident moves into the AL setting. Those lessons learned are the focus of this chapter, which recognizes that the best quality balance is one that is realistic and fits both the resident and the provider.

THE CONTEXT OF QUALITY IN AL

The residents' voices heard in the preceding chapters made it clear that standard quality indicators used by researchers or regulatory agencies, such as an increase in functional impairment or the development of pressure ulcers, are not what residents think about when considering quality in AL. To be clear, although residents *do* care about their physical and psychosocial well-being, they are focused less on outcomes and more on processes. *How* staff help them to avoid challenges such as increased impairment and pressure ulcers, for example, is most important; the staff members may accomplish this by adopting a supportive, individualized manner when caring for residents.

To understand the overall context of quality, it is necessary to listen for the overarching concepts that residents discussed when asked about what constitutes quality in AL. Much of their talk about quality fell within six domains. Residents' perceptions of quality related to (1) themselves (as intimated by Ms. Gentile); (2) home operations; (3) the physical environment; (4) the staff; (5) food and dining; and (6) social life. Table 8.1 lists these domains, with specific topics under each to indicate the nuanced and numerous dimensions within which individuals consider what they value. Each will be discussed briefly, so that

- prospective or current residents and families may consider what matters most to them, and
- providers may consider the areas in which they have strengths, as well as the areas in which change may be beneficial and is consistent with their mission and capacity.

For residents, families, and providers, though, it should be kept in mind that the diversity among individuals makes it impossible for a given setting to be all things to all people—nor should it be, in fact. AL by its very nature was developed to provide choice and allow diversity to accommodate different styles and preferences, and so moving toward a one-size-fits-all "McDonaldization" of AL is not the intent (Zimmerman & Sloane, 2007).

Quality as Related to the Self

As we see in Table 8.1, individuals vary in the extent to which they value being able to do things for themselves (control), are concerned about their physical and cognitive status (health), and reflect on whether they are spending their money wisely (money matters). Residents, families, and providers are encouraged to consider—for a given resident, in an individualized manner—which of these topics

Table 8.1. AL Residents' Perceptions of Quality:
Domains, Topics, and Examples

Domain and Topic	Description / Example
Self	
Acceptance, rejection	Need to be here, moved in at right or wrong time
Beliefs, attitudes	Political or religious beliefs, humor, philosophy; reputation of place
Control	Doing or not doing for oneself
Consumer	Being a purchaser of services, owned things
Health	Own physical and cognitive status
History	Previous experiences, expectations
Interests	Having hobbies, profession, other valued outlets
Money matters	Feelings of affordability, money being well spent
Privacy	Enough or not enough, concerns
Spending time	How time is spent, whether it is as one wishes
AL home operations	
Administrator (boss)	Quality of boss, operations, and management
Ambience	What "feels right" about the place
Maintenance	Cleanliness and repair of public and private spaces
Medical and other services	Sufficient or not
Rules, regulations, policies	Positive or negative aspects related to AL, state, or federal
Safety, security	Feelings of safety, having locks
Things to do	Offering too many or too few, things that are—or are not—of interest
Physical environment	
Accessibility	Getting around inside, wheelchairs, doors and elevators
Coming and going	Rules about leaving, availability of transportation
Furnishings	Comfort, homelike or institutional, personal possessions
Outdoors	Views and outdoor spaces
Proximity	Close to or far from family, community, church
Public spaces	Manner in which public space is used
Resident's room	Size, adequacy
Temperature	Too hot or cold, ability to regulate temperature

(continued)

Table 8.1. AL Residents' Perceptions of Quality:
Domains, Topics, and Examples (*continued*)

Domain and Topic	Description / Example
Staff	
Caring intangibles	Emotional, spiritual care, sense of community, personalized attention
Number and turnover	Staff shortages, retention
Orientation	Staff attitudes and approaches, including conveying respect
Oversight	Supervision provided, such as for fall prevention or for dementia
Responsiveness	Quick or slow response, including conveying that "it's not my job"
Training	Staff's knowledge or lack of knowledge of their jobs, including the need for more training
Food and dining	
Dining room interaction	Tables, partners, interactions with staff
Menu variety	Food options, variety, and availability
Nutrition	Meeting or not meeting nutritional and dietary restrictions
Options	Meals in room, choices of food/snacks
Preparation	Institutional food or food of a home-cooked nature
Schedule	Timing and whether service is—or is not—prompt
Social life	
Family support	Having contact with—and support of—family
Friends	Having friends or close bonds with others living here
Getting along	Positive or negative attitudes, behaviors of others
Helping others	Doing things to provide benefit to others
Other residents	Cognitive and physical function, appearance of others
Similarity	Similarity to other residents in areas, like gender, social class, education
Social contact, communication	Social interactions, comfort living with others, adequacy

is most operative if the quality balance is not optimal, and how to address it. Perhaps more control over food choice and time of eating could be achieved by stocking preferred food items in the resident's cabinet; concerns about physical status could be addressed by having a physical therapy evaluation; or reflections about money could be attended to by discussing AL charges in the context of the resident's overall finances.

Quality of the Home Operations

Some of the topics related to quality of the AL home operations are easier to address than others. For example, it is markedly easier to attend to cleanliness and repairs (maintenance) than it is to change the "feeling" of the setting (ambience). Still, all of the topics by which residents consider quality can open the door for communication and modification, particularly if the time is taken to purposefully review the seven areas in Table 8.1. In fact, compared to the next area of physical environment, it may be markedly more feasible to modify the home operations than it is to change the surroundings.

Quality of the Physical Environment

Regarding the physical environment, it may be here that the quality balance is most evident, even before a resident moves in. If there is limited space for a power wheelchair (accessibility), or restricted times during which transportation to medical appointments is available (coming and going), or no land for gardening (outdoors), then residents and families who require or value these things may be advised that quality balance may be hard to achieve. Still, a good fit in other domains may compensate for limitations in the physical environment, so quality is best considered in the totality of all domains and areas listed in Table 8.1.

Quality of the Staff

The challenges of staffing in residential long-term care settings are not new. Turnover at all levels of staff is common, and there is an insufficient number of workers to meet the needs of the population. Many residents and families are not aware that it is physically and emotionally demanding to work in a long-term care setting; that injuries and stress are common; that wages and benefits are not competitive with other jobs; and that staff may have little opportunity for advancement and may not feel respected (National Center for Health Workforce Analyses, Bureau of Health Professions, Health Resources and Services Administration, 2004). Administrators often do what they can to attract, retain, and train staff, but it tends to be an uphill battle. Resident and family education may be helpful if concerns about quality in this area (number and turnover) are raised, and novel solutions may be considered, such as augmenting the workforce with increased family involvement. There also are some tools with which staff attitudes (orientation) can be better understood and perhaps changed, such as a brief checklist that helps staff reflect on how person-centered and helpful their perspectives are when working with residents with dementia (Zimmerman et al., 2005). (Additional resources in this area may be obtained from PHINational: http://phinational.org/)

Quality of the Food and Dining Arrangements

Opinions about the quality of food are ubiquitous in long-term care settings. AL residents discussed quality in terms of menu variety, nutrition, options, preparation, and the scheduling of meals. It is worth noting, however, that such discussions may reflect matters other than the food itself. That is, food choice may well be the one area that offers the most variability in a given day, thereby lending itself to discussion; further, food is something about which all residents have a history, resulting in both expectations and true preferences; and finally, food choice intersects the important matters of individuality and autonomy. At the same time, it is important to note that residents do not necessarily rate the quality of food as worse than the quality they perceive in other areas (Gill, Williams, Zimmerman, & Uman, 2007), but instead think that it is an area that does indeed fit within the quality balance. AL providers tend to be responsive to food preferences to the extent they are able, but if a balance is hard to achieve, it may be helpful for providers, residents, and families to consider some of the areas (such as individuality and autonomy) that may be at the core of the imbalance.

Quality of Residents' Social Life

Residents also discussed quality in reference to dining room interactions, which relates to the broader category of social life. The next section ("Lessons Learned") will position social life within the context of human needs. For now, though, it is helpful to recognize that perceptions of quality relate to how similar one individual sees herself or himself as being to others, socially or in terms of health or cognition, which can certainly be noticeable, even obvious, at the time that a choice of residence is being made. At the same time, residents gain meaning from being able to help others, suggesting that residents who have reciprocal strengths—such as the wheelchair-bound Ms. Larson getting help with laundry from her more mobile, but increasingly confused, roommate, whom Ms. Larson helped to navigate daily life in AL—may perceive more quality through participating in a helping relationship. Finally, it is helpful to recognize that perceptions of quality of social life relate to the availability of family, and so an environment within which family members feel welcomed and comfortable is important to achieve balance.

THE BASIS OF QUALITY IN AL

On a deeper level, the areas within which residents frame quality are useful when considering not only what is realistic and feasible, but also how to prioritize quality improvement. Readers who have taken an introductory psychology class may remember Abraham Maslow and his concept of a "hierarchy of needs" (Maslow, 1943). The five levels of needs begin with the most basic *physiological* needs, including things such as food and sleep. Assuming those needs are satisfied, *safety* becomes of importance, including security of the self and one's possessions. Having met physiological and safety needs, those related to *love and belonging* require attention, and can be fulfilled through relationships with family and friends. The next higher level is *esteem* needs, such as confidence, achievement, and being respected by others. The highest level of need fulfillment is *self-actualization*, achieving one's highest potential. With this typology in mind, there is a clear ordering of the importance of the domains in achieving a quality balance.

Overall, few residents addressed concerns about having their *physiological needs* met; presumably, AL communities that do not fulfill these needs do not exist or if they do, are soon out of business. Mr. Guarino expressly noted that Arcadia Springs met this important need for him, as he wasn't eating properly prior to his move there. Yet, although physiological needs may be met, physiological *preferences* may not be, and it is conceivable that the line between the two may be blurred on occasion, such as when Ms. Tieman complained about the lack of strict dietary enforcement for diabetics.

Safety needs were also addressed by residents—for example, Ms. Powell, who wished for a lock on her door to ensure that her belongings were safe—but these needs seem to be primarily met and so are not a common topic of conversation in resident interviews. These two lowest levels align more closely with the "floor" of quality, which serves as the focus of attention in state regulations, noted in Chapter 6. Instead, the preponderance of discussion focused on the quality of meeting needs related to *love and belonging*, which merited an entire chapter to illustrate the importance of a culture of caring. The need for love and belonging parallels the social life domain of quality that residents discussed and also the caring intangibles related to the staff, indicating that it is an important human need that residents recognize relates to quality. It is rather fascinating to consider this finding in terms of the foundation of AL, which was built on a social model of care (Kane & Wilson, 1993). In that regard, there is a strong fit between what residents consider most important to quality and the needs that developers were seeking to fulfill. How well that goal has been achieved varies, however, as we learned from the stories shared in the preceding chapters.

The tenets of AL are also to treat residents with dignity and respect (Assisted Living Quality Coalition, 1998), which is consistent with Maslow's next highest level of needs, those related to *self-esteem*. Although some residents perceived quality in this way—such as Ms. Streeter, who said, "*I do everything,*" including bathing and medication management—there was less discussion of self-esteem than of the more basic needs. Finally, even fewer residents considered quality in the context of *self-actualization*, although it was evident when Martha St. John felt accomplishment and purpose from her range of activities as "morale officer" at Boxwood Gardens. Overall, however, residents perceive the AL's role in creating quality as related to their being physiologically sound, safe, having a sense of belonging, and maintaining their self-esteem. Although a wish for self-actualization remains, AL residents do not seem to hold the setting responsible for helping them achieve this highest potential.

LESSONS LEARNED AND STRATEGIES TO ACHIEVE A QUALITY BALANCE

Considering the context and basis of quality may be a helpful orienting framework for providers, as is the ultimate importance of *person–environment fit* (Lawton & Nahemow, 1975), which was introduced in Chapter 1. The challenge of fit is that each individual is different, of course, and one setting cannot be expected to be all things to all people. However, resident variability provides guidance for providers, as do these observations gleaned from earlier chapters:

- Residents have preconceived expectations of quality. As Jean Thompson told us, Murray Ridge was *"pretty much what [she] thought it would be,"* based on the fact that her cousin had previously lived there. Jean also had had prior experiences in nursing homes, which influenced her frame of reference.
  Lesson learned: Attend to perceptions of quality before move-in.
- Residents change their perceptions of what constitutes quality over time. Jean also talked about having to become adjusted to her dependence on staff, suggesting that staff availability was initially less important but became more so with time.
  Lesson learned: Attend to perceptions of quality over time.
- Residents differ in their perceptions of what constitutes quality. Jean Thompson, Millie Fischer, and Eileen Howe all lived in Murray Ridge, yet each talked about quality differently. Jean commented on individuality; Millie focused on the absence of her family; and Eileen noted the lack of an institutional feel.
  Lesson learned: Attend to each individual's perception of quality.
- Residents don't always share their perceptions of quality. We heard Ms. Bachman not want to voice her complaints about St. Brigid AL, because *"They'd probably throw you out,"* even though she was not aware of that ever happening. Indeed, residents are dependent on staff, and although we heard virtually no reports or concerns of neglect or abuse, the drive to remain in the good graces of a caregiver is a strong one.
  Lesson learned: Actively solicit perceptions of quality.
- Residents' families' perceptions of quality may be at odds with residents' own perceptions. As if the complexity of quality weren't

already sufficient, family members have their own perceptions. Ms. Hebel, aware of and able to express her preference for no nightly room checks, found her wishes ranked by the AL management below her daughter's preference to keep them (Morgan, 2009). Further, we heard and witnessed cases wherein families have control and authority even when there is no formal power of attorney in place to exert it.
Lesson learned: Solicit and attend to families' perceptions of quality, both before move-in and over time.

- Staff perceptions of quality may be at odds with those of residents and families. Staff may not recognize as important the same things that residents and families find important, as was the case with Donna, the care aide who preferred that residents not have locks on their doors because it impeded safety—although we know Ms. Powell, among others, preferred locks (Morgan, 2009). Similar observations have been made in nursing homes, where, for example, staff underestimate the importance residents put on contact with the outside world and overestimate the importance they place on activities and food (Kane et al., 1997). This disconnect is especially important because staff are the ultimate conduit of quality in AL. Even residents who value the physical environment found it to be of secondary importance to their relationships with staff.
Lesson learned: Involve staff in discussions of resident and family perceptions of quality before move-in and over time; solicit staff members' own perceptions at the time of hiring and over time; and reduce the disconnect between their perceptions and those of residents and families.

- Perceptions of quality may be—or may appear to be—at odds with regulations. Food is an area in which regulations (at least in part) result in meals that are not always to residents' liking. If these same individuals were living independently, their choice of meals would not be bound by such restrictions, but meals also might not be as nutritious. Although it is not uncommon to offer more than one meal option—and in some cases buffets are available—accommodating residents' preferences will, at least on occasion, result in food choices that are perceived to be of poor quality by the staff.
Lesson learned: Within the bounds of regulations, be creative in seeking solutions to maximize quality.

Table 8.2 summarizes these lessons learned and provides examples of actions to take to attend to and promote a quality balance in assisted living.

Table 8.2. Lessons Learned: Strategies to Achieve a Quality Balance

Lesson Learned	Example/Action
Attend to perceptions of quality before move-in	Using the domains and areas presented earlier, ask what a prospective resident and his or her family members desire and expect, and be specific and realistic in discussing the extent to which their desires can be met.
	• Don't promise what cannot be delivered, and do recognize that "one size does not fit all" may affect the bottom line—meaning not all communities will be suitable for a given individual, and not all individuals will be suitable for a given community.
	• The goodness of fit is more than the ability to attend to necessary "care" needs; instead, it should be based on the ability to attend to different "quality" needs.
	• Being up-front about the quality balance will allow prospective residents and their families to differentiate one setting from another, and also help certain settings stand apart from others.
Attend to perceptions of quality over time	Individuals' needs change, especially when they are older adults, who can be expected to require more services and support over time. At the same time, characteristics of the AL setting change, sometimes by design (such as when new activities are introduced) and sometimes by default (such as when the overall cohort of residents ages).
	• Resident councils and committees are increasingly commonplace in AL as a strategy to air perceptions of quality, but if such meetings focus on areas needing improvement, it may be human nature for leadership to become defensive and for residents to then become angry or feel powerless.
	• There is a power differential in AL, and although the residents and families are the customers, they are dependent on the administration; for this reason, residents may not feel comfortable openly airing their concerns.
	• Bringing in an outsider to serve as a facilitator, such a staff member from another AL residence, may help assure that both parties feel comfortable and understand each other when discussing the quality balance.

(continued)

Table 8.2. Lessons Learned: Strategies to Achieve a
Quality Balance *(continued)*

Lesson Learned	Example/Action
Attend to each individual's perception of quality	Because quality means different things to different people, it may be helpful to consider the different domains and areas summarized earlier (Table 8.1) when considering the quality balance: self, home operations, physical environment, staff, food and dining, and social life. • Although in some cases it will be challenging to please residents who are diametrically opposed in their perceptions as to what constitutes quality, assuring fit at the time of move-in will help to moderate differences between residents. • No more than moderate differences between residents will promote their social life, and the importance of a social life for AL residents cannot be overstated.
Actively solicit perceptions of quality	Individual differences mean that some residents will be vocal in their opinions and others will not be. • Similar to resident councils and committees, consumer satisfaction surveys have become commonplace in AL to solicit feedback, but they do not typically address all areas considered by residents to be important in the quality balance. Also, even surveys developed by experts may be worded in such a way as to solicit positive responses. • If one really wants to promote a better quality balance, it will be more beneficial to ask "What can be done to make you feel more secure here?" than it is to ask "On a scale of 1–4, how secure do you feel here?" • At the same time, the power differential may make it unsafe to share feelings in other than an anonymous manner, which makes it impossible to know which residents are feeling which ways. • Over time, however, active solicitation and responsiveness will make for a better quality balance and an environment in which differences can be openly discussed.

(continued)

224

Table 8.2.   Lessons Learned: Strategies to Achieve a
Quality Balance   *(continued)*

Lesson Learned	Example/Action
Solicit and attend to families' perceptions of quality before move-in and over time	At any given time, there are as many AL customers as there are residents and their involved family members, and all of them may differently weigh domains and areas of the quality balance. • When multiple parties are involved, special skills may be needed to negotiate differences, such as those of a social worker who can be brought in on a consulting basis. Short of working through such differences, though, all actions noted above in this table are relevant to family members, including attending to and actively soliciting their perceptions of quality before move-in and over time.
Involve staff in discussions of resident's and family's perceptions of quality before move-in and over time; solicit staff's own perceptions at the time of hiring and over time; reduce the disconnect between staff's perceptions and those of residents and families	The final constituency involved in the quality balance is the staff, and, as with residents and families, they too are individuals who weigh domains and areas differently. Further, together with the residents, they live the balance on a daily basis. Although the importance of staff as those who know the residents best is now recognized, their special knowledge is not typically capitalized upon; that is, although they may become involved when a problem needs attention, their expertise is not often solicited in advance to proactively discuss their understanding of the residents' and family members' perceptions of quality. • Tasking staff with the roles of "quality experts" will both recognize their importance and bring to the forefront areas of disconnect that can then be addressed.

(continued)

Table 8.2.   Lessons Learned: Strategies to Achieve a
Quality Balance   *(continued)*

Lesson Learned	Example/Action
Within the bounds of regulations, be creative in seeking solutions to maximize quality	By their very intent, regulations are intended to promote quality, but at the same time they set parameters that dictate the nature of the setting, the services that can be provided, and the residents who can be accommodated. Still, few of the domains and areas within which residents think of quality are counter to regulations, and so the matter herein is the mindset of saying "yes" and seeking solutions to promote the quality balance.
	• AL providers typically meet with their peers and attend local, regional, and national meetings at which innovations in care are discussed.
	• Some of this information might be brought back to residents, families, and staff, which would serve the dual purpose of having all recognize that quality is a consistent focus and allowing all to weigh in on new strategies to promote the quality balance.

The actions described and the messages of this chapter—
which are based on the words of AL residents conveyed in earlier
chapters—are not meant to suggest that one should *expect* imbalance
in the quality of fit or look for things that are *wrong*. Further, it truly
is the *fit* between the resident and the setting that determine quality,
not characteristics of one in isolation of the other. For example, when
asked to apply an overall grade to their setting, the two settings that
received the best grades were the one that was the most expensive
(Winter Hills) and the one with the lowest charges (St. Brigid). They
catered to different clientele, with Winter Hills being described with
words such as *"luxury"* or *"my God, it's beautiful—it's like a bed and
breakfast,"* while residents at St. Brigid spoke of the importance of
"big windows" and it being *"a tremendous blessing we have the Chapel
right there."*

Two common threads that made these settings similar were that
both had a strong, consistent, and evident philosophy that guided

daily interactions between staff and residents, and that in both there was a core of staff members who had been there for a long while and who "go the extra mile" for those residing there. In Winter Hills, "residents' rights are first and foremost...when a new employee is hired they learn very quickly that the residents come first." Of St. Brigid, Mr. Grier said, *"As senile as we could be, we're always right...as far as I'm concerned, I could not speak enough about the goodness in this place here."*

Thus, once again, if one were to identify the *most* important component within the quality balance, it seems to be that of the caring intangibles and the social life, of meeting the human need for love and belonging (Eckert, Zimmerman, & Morgan, 2001). In Winter Hills, Mrs. Braun's niece described the moment of her death by saying "I turned around when she died, and they [the staff] were just all tears...they were all there, and that said a lot to me." Indeed, the lesson most learned is that quality balance is achieved through relationships, one person to another, and that it is both feasible and evident in AL.

REFERENCES

Assisted Living Quality Coalition. (1998). *Assisted living quality initiative. Building a structure that promotes quality.* Washington, DC: Public Policy Institute, American Association of Retired Persons.

Eckert, J. K., Zimmerman, S. I., & Morgan, L. A. (2001). Connectedness in assisted living: A qualitative perspective. In S. I. Zimmerman, P. Sloane, & J. K. Eckert (Eds.), *Assisted living: Residential care in transition* (pp. 292–316). Baltimore, MD: Johns Hopkins University Press.

Gill, K. S., Williams, C. S., Zimmerman, S., & Uman, G. (2007). Quality of long-term care as reported by residents with dementia. *Alzheimer's Care Today, 8*(4), 344–358.

Kane, R., & Wilson, K. B., (Eds.). (1993). *Assisted living in the United States: A new paradigm for residential care for frail older persons?* Washington, DC: Public Policy Institute, American Association of Retired Persons.

Kane, R. A., Caplan, A. L., Urv-Wong, E. K., Freeman, I. C., Aroskar, M. A., & Finch, F. (1997). Everyday matters in the lives of nursing home residents: Wish for and perception of choice and control. *Journal of the American Geriatrics Society, 45,* 1086–1093.

Lawton, M. P., & Nahemow, L. (1975). Ecology and the aging process. In C. Eisdorfer & M. P. Lawton (Eds.), *Psychology of adult development and aging.* Washington, DC: American Psychological Association.

Maslow, A. H. (1943). A theory of human motivation. *Psychological Review, 50*(4), 370–396.

Morgan, L. A. (2009). Balancing safety and privacy: The case of room locks in assisted living. *Journal of Housing for the Elderly, 23*(3), 185–203.

National Center for Health Workforce Analyses, Bureau of Health Professions, Health Resources and Services Administration. (2004). Nursing aides, home health aides, and related health care occupations—National and local workforce shortages and associated data needs. Retrieved from ftp://ftp.hrsa.gov/bhpr/nationalcenter/RNandHomeAides.pdf

Seligman, M. E. P. (1975). *Helplessness: On depression, development, and death.* San Francisco, CA: W.H. Freeman.

Zimmerman, S., & Sloane, P. D. (2007). Definition and classification of assisted living. *The Gerontologist, 47*(6), 33–39.

Zimmerman, S., Williams, C. S., Reed, P. S., Boustani, M., Preisser, J. S., Heck, E., & Sloane, P. D. (2005). Attitudes, stress and satisfaction of staff caring for residents with dementia [Special issue]. *The Gerontologist, 45*(1), 96–105.

Appendix
Research Methods Used for the Study

The bulk of the information employed in this book derives from a 4-year research study entitled "Stakeholders' Models of Quality in Assisted Living," funded by the National Institute on Aging (L. A. Morgan, Principal Investigator). The goal of the project was to contact residents in diverse assisted living (AL) settings to determine their views, and those of their kin, direct care staff, and managers/directors working in these settings, about the concepts upon which their evaluations of quality are based. Based on earlier research, we had reason to expect that, while everyone talked about quality, perhaps they did not all mean the same thing.

Using mixed methods, the study included both semi-structured interviews and a more numerically oriented card-sorting step, described in the section on Data Collection Techniques later in this Appendix. The intention of the study's design was not to represent the entire population of AL settings, residents, or other participants (including family and staff). Instead, the goal of the study was to "drill down" to gain a grounded understanding of what matters most in AL, including the criteria upon which the participants in these settings make their judgments of quality. Here, we focus most centrally on the views of residents. The study's aims were as follows:

1. To elicit and describe the essential elements of the meaning of *quality* from the AL residents' point of view.
2. To examine variation in these meanings among residents by functional status, gender, tenure in AL, and race/ethnicity.
3. To examine the meanings of quality in other stakeholder groups (i.e., AL administrators, direct care staff, and resident families) through:
    (a) interviews to elicit elements of AL resident quality from other stakeholder groups' perspectives
    (b) prioritizing elements of quality derived from the residents' narratives

4. To have AL residents determine (via card sort) the extent to which elements attached to their definitions of quality were commensurate with those emerging from other stakeholder groups.

SETTING SAMPLE

Given that the intended sample of nine AL settings was reduced to seven due to a reduction in the budget, it became especially important to seek participation from AL settings that represented the diversity of environments in that sector. Because the project design called for a minimum of 10 residents to be interviewed in each setting, we ruled out using the "small" settings (under 16 residents) from the Collaborative Studies of Long-Term Care (CS-LTC) sampling frame (Zimmerman, Sloane, & Eckert, 2001), which was employed for this project. Among the remaining "traditional" and "new model" settings, we identified all AL facilities within 30 miles of our campus that had not been involved in multiple recent studies related to the CS-LTC, to avoid "research site burnout." This generated 166 potentially eligible AL settings. We examined several parameters of variation widely used in research, with a goal of intentionally identifying those that would provide diversity with respect to location in terms of urban/suburban/rural areas; chain/independent ownership; for-profit or nonprofit status; religious/nonreligious sponsorship; and number of residents, their racial/ethnic composition, socioeconomic status, and percent with notable dementia. (See Table 1.1 in Chapter 1 for a list of selected sites.)

After targeting a subset of the eligible AL settings, we began to identify those willing to participate. We rejected three sites because of very high rates of residents with dementia, which would make it difficult to obtain enough interviews from this group. Four sites turned us down for reasons including incomplete leadership/management transitions, being engaged in other research, or corporate opposition. As sites were eliminated, we identified alternates that captured the traits of diversity. Our strategy generated a group of AL settings that represent diversity on key setting-level traits.

GAINING ACCESS

In making contact and gaining access to the AL sites, we used the same successful strategy we had used in the "Transitions from Assisted Living

Study" (Eckert, Carder, Morgan, Frankowski, & Roth, 2009; J.K. Eckert, Principal Investigator). Initial contact was made via phone call to the executive director or similar senior manager to determine willingness to participate. The project offered AL settings a $2,500 honorarium for their agreement to participate, with the understanding that they could withdraw at any time during research and retain these funds. A positive initial reaction was followed by a face-to-face meeting between the executive director/manager, the study PI, and the assigned researcher, who would be conducting interviews in that setting. At this meeting, the phases of the study were explained, any questions answered, and information necessary to process the honorarium was collected.

Participating AL settings were invited to make use of the honorarium dollars to benefit their residents, with the choice of how to use this money left to their discretion. At one site it was used to purchase new patio furniture for a renovated outdoor area; in another it was used for a sound system and in a third for a catered dinner for staff and residents. Participants were interested in the study and hearing about the findings. Support of the executive directors involved notifying the staff and residents about the study, agreeing to assist the researchers in identifying residents who might be appropriate for interview, and introducing the researcher to others in the setting. Their ongoing support was vital to successful completion of the work.

SAMPLING PERSONS WITHIN SETTINGS

Resident Sample

Once the AL settings were on board, the next step was to identify and recruit residents to participate in semi-structured interviews, focusing on their experiences of daily life in AL. We sought to complete 10 resident interviews in each of the 7 settings. The researchers assigned to each site worked with managers and members of the staff, such as activities personnel and others, to identify potential participants capable of interview. One goal of the study was to include, if possible, residents with mild cognitive impairment. Given the significant percentage of those with Alzheimer's disease or other forms of dementia in AL, including the views of this group adds a broader resident perspective, important in the understanding of AL today. Clearly some residents were not cognitively able to be interviewed, and some interviews were of limited value in attempting to meet this goal of bringing in perspectives of those with dementia (see the discussion in the following section on Family, Staff, and Manager Interviews for more information regarding this point).

It was then up to the researchers in each site to make contact with residents, explain the study, gain informed consent, and conduct interviews. Interviews included a description of how the person came to live in the setting and a range of questions intended to identify the specific factors that shaped their experience of quality in their AL, regardless of whether it was positive, mixed, or negative. The interview guide, used with some flexibility by the researcher, is attached to this appendix. Interviews ranged from 20 to 120 minutes and were tape recorded. In some instances interviews required two visits, due to daily schedules (e.g., mealtimes) or other interruptions. Interviews covered a wide array of topics, with some residents focusing their comments on problems or issues in the environment, others lauding the performance of personnel and leadership of their setting, or providing nuanced, mixed pictures of both positive and negative aspects of daily life. Our focus in these interviews was not to determine a resident's evaluation of the setting (although a question to that effect was included toward the end of the interview), but rather to determine upon what areas (e.g., food, staff attitudes, room amenities, location, etc.) and specific elements within these (e.g., food's nutrition or menu variety) mattered more in their evaluative frameworks. Whereas some interviews range across a wide array of topics, other residents focus on a single theme or topic, sometimes in considerable depth.

Family, Staff, and Manager Interviews

The study also called for interviews of three other stakeholder groups: family members of residents (relatives of those we interviewed, if possible, plus two family members for residents with moderate to severe dementia, who themselves were unable to participate in interviews, N = 12), and five members of the direct care staff (to include hands-on care providers, select members of the dining, housekeeping, and laundry staff and others, such as medication staff) with regular, meaningful interactions with residents. In addition, we sought to interview three management/administrative staff, ideally to include the executive director and two additional administrators/managers. Given the diversity among the sites in the study, lines between "direct care" and "management" were not entirely consistent or clear across facilities (e.g., an activities director might be treated as management at one site and elsewhere be closer to the level of a direct care provider). Consequently, the researchers were asked to make judgment calls, based on their experiences in these settings, as to how to categorize and consider these employees for interviewing purposes. All interviewees were selected to have a minimum of 6 months in the setting, be currently employed there, and at least have regular daily contact with residents.

These management/staff definitions also came into play regarding the incentives we offered to direct care workers. Our intention was to provide incentives to the lower-paid and time-challenged direct care staff members, who might need to meet with our researcher team member for interviews outside their standard working hours. The sites varied in their reactions to the appropriateness of these incentives, and we responded according to their traditions and policies with regard to interviews on "company time" and the provision of these $25 gift card to the direct care staff.

In a similar vein, we took our cues from the management of each AL site with regard to the appropriate means to contact the relatives of residents about participating in the study, as described below. Sometimes contacts were made directly within the AL setting, but other managers preferred to send letters to all responsible kin or take another approach. In all groups, we intended to select participants who would provide diverse views.

DATA COLLECTION TECHNIQUES AND PHASING OF THE STUDY

Data Collection Techniques

Two distinct approaches to data collection are combined in this study. First, as discussed earlier, semi-structured interviews, tape recorded and transcribed for analysis, comprise one major component. All residents, family members, staff, and managers were involved in parallel, semi-structured interviews. Some additional data were collected in the interviews, including physical functioning ratings (using the ADL scale) for residents (self-ratings by the residents and proxy ratings by kin); managers completed a set of additional questions regarding the setting and its operations. All participants gave verbal consent on tape for their involvement, and all taped interviews were transcribed and thematically coded, as described later.

The second data collection technique involved a structured card sorting task. All four groups participated in card sorting, but the exact cards included in the sort and timing of this task differed for the groups, as will be discussed in the next section. Each person was provided a set of laminated cards with statements about AL, describing a trait that emerged from our analysis of interviews. The cards carried a meaningless identification number on the back, simply used to record the results of the card sort quickly following administration. Initially, the participants are asked to take the cards and sort them into two piles: one pile contains items that the person sorting considered to be "important" or to "matter" in AL. In the case of family members, the instructions make the task personal, focusing on their relative. For residents, the task focuses on what matters/is important to them. Staff and managers were asked to sort the cards based on what matters/is important to residents in general. The instructions emphasize that they are not being asked to rate whether the AL does the task well or poorly—only whether the item described on the card is important to themselves, to their relative, or to residents in general, depending on the respondent's role.

Once this initial sorting is complete, with prompts/reminders of the task as necessary and the option of revisiting and moving cards from one stack to the other, the cards identified as "not important" are discarded. Sorters are then asked to take all of the "important" cards and conduct a second sort to identify those items that are the "most important" among them. For each of these sorts, no specific number of cards was required in any given pile, but sorters are encouraged to have at least some cards in each pile. At the end of the sorting, the piles are collected and the results are recorded by card number.

The card sorting process was also tape recorded to capture any useful commentary by the sorters as they consider the items on the cards. Pilot testing of the card sort process indicated that residents took considerably longer than the other three groups to complete the task, and that prompts from researchers, as well as visual prompts on a sorting board to remind them of the "important/matters" theme of the task are essential to ensuring that the sort is conducted as intended. Transcripts were informative methodologically in clarifying how well this task actually worked in the field. Whereas most participants in the other three groups completed the card sorting task without problem, quite a few residents had difficulty in—or declined to—complete this task, particularly the second step of determining which items were most important, resulting in limited usefulness of these data across groups.

Phasing of the Study

The data collection for this study was conducted in three major phases:

1. Resident interviews were conducted in the initial phase. These interviews provided the basic data for developing the initial coding categories through a team coding process, described later. This process developed approximately 54 coding categories that reflect elements of quality and related topics that we wish to retrieve/analyze from the narrative database. The quality-related code constructs were the basis for development of the initial set of cards, used in the card sort process for staff, managers, and family members.

2. Family, staff, and manager data collection. This second phase involved conducting both the semi-structured interviews and the card sorting task in a single visit for all three nonresident groups. Each participant was asked to complete the interview, identifying elements that serve as the basis of their assessments of quality, as well as any other data collection needed (e.g., setting information for managers, ADL evaluation from family members, and demographic information for all respondents). All participants in these groups were then asked to complete the card sorting process described earlier, using cards based on the concepts that had emerged from resident interviews.

Following these interviews, another round of team coding occurred, adding a few more coding categories for different themes that emerged from the interviews with the other three groups. These themes were subsequently turned into cards to be sorted in Phase 3.

3. Resident card sorting. Once the concepts/themes from all four groups had been identified and converted into cards, we returned again to meet with the remaining (or replacement) residents for the card sorting step of data collection. The sorting task was the same as it had been for the other groups, only the card deck for residents included a few concepts added in the second phase of the project, reflecting family, staff, and management priorities. Again, the sorting process was taped, with any commentary transcribed to become part of the database. Responses to the cards, including stories of noteworthy positive or negative quality experiences, were deemed valuable additions to the database.

DATA MANAGEMENT AND ANALYSIS

Collaborative Coding Process

Development and refinement of coding categories for these data was a thought-provoking and time-consuming task. It began with detailed reading of a limited number of interviews by all members of the research team, with regular meetings to discuss concepts that individuals on the team saw emerging from the interviews. Several sets of interviews were reviewed via this collaborative process, gradually building an initial list of emergent themes, which were tested and retested against additional interviews until a preliminary list of codes took form. This coding list remained provisional for a period of months, as additional interviews were examined in relation to the team's capacity to code meaningful content using it. Eventually, a consensus set of codes emerged that could be used, along with memos and other coding techniques, to annotate the interviews in the narrative database.

Once the code list was essentially complete, coding the interviews and fieldnotes began, with rotating, two-person teams assigned materials to code individually. Coding reconciliation sessions permitted these teams to discuss their application of the codes, leading to further refinement of how the codes were defined and applied. This process continued, with ongoing feedback in biweekly meetings, until the entire set of interviews, and associated fieldnotes, were coded.

The coded information is maintained in a database using the Atlas-ti qualitative software package (Scientific Software Development, 2007). This software has a broad capacity to search, associate, and assist in theory development and testing in the large database generated by this project. With this completed database, the research team can search for content about particular sites in the study, subgroups (such as family members), or use individual codes or combinations of codes to identify all narrative related to a theme or topic of interest.

Analysis

Strategies for analysis used in this book varied somewhat across chapters and topics covered. For example, we made only very limited use of the card sort data here. Our primary focus was to search for evidence regarding residents' meanings related to quality within the narrative database. Often the searches focused on single codes or series of related codes from 50+ coding categories (see code list in Chapter 8). There were select codes, for example, that pertained most clearly to Chapter 3, including "staff orientations" and "caregiving intangibles," intended to capture experiences relevant to the culture of care within AL. In other cases, analysis focused on answers to particular questions within a subgroup, such as answers to the "what makes a good day?" question among residents, which served as a substantial basis for views on, and variations in, quality criteria described in Chapter 1. In other cases, searches were made by several code categories (e.g., Chapter 4 on food) or use of varied groups' voices, as in the chapters on regulation and change in AL (Chapters 6 and 7), where voices of staff and managers in AL augmented those of residents and their family members. Use of filters, for example, to consider only the interviews with residents, were combined with searches on single or multiple codes to target desired content. Construction of all chapters involved input of multiple members of the research team.

QUALITY INTERVIEW GUIDE

Resident/Family Interview

We are interested in learning more about what things are important to the residents here in their everyday lives.

After reviewing the informed consent information sheet, turn on the tape recorder and ask "Is it okay to go ahead with the interview and tape record it?"

Background

1. When did you move to this setting/place?
2. Tell me about the events that led to you coming to live here.
3. How did this place get selected? Who was involved in deciding?
4. Where had you lived prior to coming here?
5. (If appropriate to follow-up) What was your experience in other AL or rehab settings?
6. Have you been in or visited other people in assisted living before? What was that like?

Resident/Quality

7. What did you expect this place to be like before you moved here?
   How is it different from what you expected?
8. On a day like today, what things make it a good day for you?
   How about a not-so-good day?
9. Tell me about what things have been important to you in your life?
   Have those things changed? How?
   Does living here make a difference in who you are and how you spend your time?

10. What things do you like about this place? What things don't you like?

11. If someone you knew was thinking about moving into assisted living, what would you tell them to look for or to avoid?

12. If you were the administrator running this place, what would you change to make life better or nicer for the people who live here? What would you leave the same?

13. Let's pretend that we are building a new place to live and you're part of the planning team.

    What should we be sure to include or do there to make residents happy?

    What things should we avoid?

    What things that are done here would you like to see included there?

14. Tell me about the other people. What kinds of things do they talk about?

    How do people get along? Are people friendly?

    How do residents and staff get along? Are there romances?

15. Are there other important things about living here that you'd like to add?

16. Is this a quality place? Why? Why not?

17. If you were to give this place a grade, what grade would you give it and why?

REFERENCES

Eckert, J. K., Carder, P. C., Morgan, L. A., Frankowski, A. C., & Roth, E. G. (2009). *Inside assisted living: The search for home.* Baltimore, MD: Johns Hopkins University Press.

Scientific Software Development. (2007). Atlas.ti 5.2.8, Retrieved from http://www.atlasti.com.

Zimmerman, S., Sloane, P. D., & Eckert, J. K. (2001). *Assisted living: Needs, practices and policies in residential care for the elderly.* Baltimore, MD: Johns Hopkins University Press.

Index

at the Greenbriar, 33–36
and interaction, 106–107, 115, 119,
121, 217–218
as microcosm, 36
multiple seatings in, 109
physical appearance of, 103–106
as soft institution, 107–110
Direct care staff, 24, 28, 67, 85. *See
also* Staff(ing)
attitudes and behaviors of,
17, 68
interaction with residents, 57–58,
70–73

Economic difficulties associated
with assisted living, 199–201
Emotional care, 58, 60, 64, 65, 69,
74, 81. *See also* Care
End-of-life care, 24, 57–60, 62, 65, 87.
See also Care

Family(ies)
dysfunctional, 35
and healthy eating, 93–94
language and cultural differences,
75–77
Fear of retaliation, residents',
142–144
Federal Interagency Forum on
Aging-Related Statistics, 92
Financial constraints, of rules and
regulations on AL, 174–177
Food, 89–122. *See also* Dining;
Healthy eating
preferences of, 95–96
preparation, institutional,
96–99
quality as related to, 214, 217
resident activist and, 89–92
Freedom to come and go,
131–134

Groups' perspectives, on
quality, 25

Health changes in residents, 185–188.
See also Change(s)
perceptions of, 186–188
unexpected, 186
Health Insurance Portability and
Accountability Act (HIPAA),
172–174
Healthy eating, 92–95. *See also*
Dining; Food
Home operations, and quality, 213, 216
Hospice care, 65. *See also* Care
Human interaction, 63–64

Independence, 51, 54
Inmate culture, 38
Institution
definition of, 37
soft, 33–55
total, 37–38, 44
Institutional life, in assisted living,
37–53. *See also* Soft institution

Language differences, between
staff and residents, 36,
75–77, 105, 196
Leadership
changes in, 190–192
corporate, 164, 192
single, 8
style, 26, 86, 164, 184, 190
Learned helplessness, 212
Level of care, changes in, 169–171
Licensed practical nurse (LPN),
166, 168

Managers. *See also* Administrators
fear of litigation, 149
leadership style, 190–192
Maslow's hierarchy of needs,
218–219
Medicaid, 174–177
Medical dimension of soft
institution, 49–50
Money, 105, 154, 174–177

Staff(ing)   (*Continued*)
scheduling duties, 72–73
training for, 73–75
turnover, 71, 197–198
well-being, 85
"Stakeholders' Models of Quality in
Assisted Living"
collaborative coding process,
236–237
data analysis, 237–238
data collection techniques,
233–236
phases of, 235–236
gaining access to AL sites,
230–231
goal of, 229
sampling persons within
settings, 231
direct care staff, 232

family members of
residents, 232
management/administrative
staff, 232–233
resident sample, 231–232
setting sample, 230
State regulations, 155–163
compared to nursing home,
158–163
quality of, 155–157
Sugar use, and autonomy,
134–136
Surveys, customer satisfaction, 5, 26,
158, 164

Training, staff, 73–75, 193, 195

Veterans Administration (VA)
Aid and Assistance, 174